INFANT STIMULATION

Summary Publications in the Johnson & Johnson Baby Products Company
Pediatric Round Table Series:

1. *Maternal Attachment and Mothering Disorders: A Round Table*
   Edited by Marshall H. Klaus, M.D.
             Treville Leger and
             Mary Anne Trause, Ph.D.

2. *Social Responsiveness of Infants*
   Edited by Evelyn B. Thoman, Ph.D. and
             Sharland Trotter

3. *Learning Through Play*
   By Paul Chance, Ph.D.

4. *The Communication Game*
   Edited by Abigail Peterson Reilly, Ph.D.

5. *Infants At Risk: Assessment and Intervention*
   Edited by Catherine Caldwell Brown

6. *Birth, Interaction and Attachment*
   Edited by Marshall Klaus, M.D. and
             Martha Oschrin Robertson

7. Minimizing High-Risk Parenting
   Edited by Valerie Sasserath, Ph.D. and
             Robert A. Hoekelman, M.D.

8. *Child Health Care Communications*
   Edited by Susan M. Thornton, M.S. and
             William K. Frankenburg, M.D.

9. *Childhood Learning Disabilities and Prenatal Risk*
   Edited by Catherine Caldwell Brown

10. *The Many Facets of Touch*
    Edited by Catherine Caldwell Brown

11. *Play Interactions: The Role of Toys and Parental Involvement in Children's Development*
    Edited by Catherine Caldwell Brown and
              Allen W. Gottfried, Ph.D.

12. *Group Care for Young Children: Considerations for Child Care and Health Professionals, Public Policy Makers, and Parents*
    Edited by Nina Gunzenhauser and
              Bettye M. Caldwell, Ph.D.

13. *Infant Stimulation: For Whom, What Kind, When, and How Much?*
    Edited by Nina Gunzenhauser

INFANT STIMULATION: FOR WHOM, WHAT KIND, WHEN, AND HOW MUCH?

Edited by
Nina Gunzenhauser

Introduction by
Edward Tronick, Ph.D.
and
Barry M. Lester, Ph.D.

Sponsored by

Johnson & Johnson
BABY PRODUCTS COMPANY

Library of Congress Cataloging in Publication Data
Main entry under title:

Infant Stimulation: For Whom, What Kind, When, and How Much?

(Johnson & Johnson Baby Products Company pediatric round table series; 13)

Summary of a conference held Oct. 1986 in Biscayne Bay, Fla.

Includes bibliography.
1. Infants (Premature) — Care — Congresses. 2. Sensory stimulation — Congresses. 3. Infants — Development — Congresses. I. Gunzenhauser, Nina. II. Johnson & Johnson Baby Products Company. III. Series. [DNLM: 1. Infant, Premature — growth & development — Congresses. 2. Physical Stimulation — in infancy & childhood — Congresses. WS 410 I43 1986]

RJ250.I54   1987   618.92'011   87-3519

ISBN 0-931562-15-5

Cover: Edward Tronick, Ph.D., Donna Drake, R.N., Barry M. Lester, Ph.D., Women & Infants Hospital of Rhode Island

Cover photo: David Whitbeck

To Robert B. Rock, Jr.

For his insight, initiative, and dedication
in making possible this publication
and the entire Pediatric Round Table Series

CONTENTS

List of Participants — ix

Preface
Robert B. Rock, Jr., M.A., M.P.A. — xi

Introduction
Barry M. Lester, Ph.D., and Edward Tronick, Ph.D. — xiii

Prologue
Edward Tronick, Ph.D. — xv

PART I—BRAIN PLASTICITY

A Comparison of Plasticity in Sensory and
Cognitive Processing Systems
Jennifer S. Buchwald, Ph.D. — 3

Brain Plasticity After Damage
Robert L. Isaacson, Ph.D. — 12

Plasticity Triggering Experiences, Nature, and the
Dual Genesis of Brain Structure and Function
D. Nico Spinelli, M.D. — 21

Development and Plasticity of the Association Cortex
Michael L. Schwartz, Ph.D., and
Patricia Goldman-Rakic, Ph.D. — 30

PART II—STIMULATION: PSYCHOLOGICAL AND
BEHAVIORAL PERSPECTIVES

Handling Preterm Infants in Hospitals: Stimulating
Controversy About Timing Stimulation
Peter A. Gorski, M.D., Lee Huntington, Ph.D., and
David J. Lewkowicz, Ph.D. — 43

State Organization in Preterm Infants: Microanalysis
of 24-Hour Polygraphic Recordings
James A. Garbanati, Ph.D., and Arthur Parmelee, M.D. — 51

Behavioral Responsivity in Preterm Infants
Cynthia Garcia Coll, Ph.D., Laura Emmons, B.A., and
Laurie Anderson, R.N., M.S. — 64

Behavioral Organization of the Newborn Preterm Infant: 71
Apathetic Organization May Not Be Abnormal
Edward Tronick, Ph.D., Kathleen B. Scanlon, M.S.N.,
and John W. Scanlon, M.D.

Behavioral and Psychophysiological   81
Assessment of the Preterm Infant
Barry M. Lester, Ph.D.

Infant Stimulation: Issues of Theory and Research   88
Anneliese F. Korner, Ph.D.

Targeting Infant Stimulation Efforts: Theoretical   97
Challenges for Research and Intervention
Frances Degen Horowitz, Ph.D.

PART III—INTERVENTION

Infants on Acute Care Hospital Units: Issues in   111
Stimulation and Intervention
Joy Goldberger, M.S.

Alleviating Stress in ICU Neonates   121
Tiffany Field, Ph.D.

Paradigms for Intervention: Infant State Modulation   129
Kathryn E. Barnard, R.N., Ph.D.

Parental Stimulation of High-Risk Infants   136
in Naturalistic Settings
Peter M. Vietze, Ph.D.

The Mother-Infant Transaction Program: An Intervention   144
for the Mothers of Low-Birthweight Infants
Virginia A. Rauh, Sc.D.,
Barry Nurcombe, M.D., F.R.A.C.P.,
Thomas Achenbach, Ph.D., and Catherine Howell, Ph.D.

Early Intervention: What Does It Mean?   157
T. Berry Brazelton, M.D.

Early Intervention: Why, For Whom, How, At What Cost?   170
Craig T. Ramey, Ph.D., Donna M. Bryant, Ph.D., and
Tanya M. Suarez, Ph.D.

Appendix: Guidelines for Stimulation of Preterm Infants   181

References   187

PARTICIPANTS

Catherine M. Balkunow
Marketing Communications
Johnson & Johnson Baby Products
  Company
Grandview Road
Skillman, New Jersey 08558

Kathryn E. Barnard, R.N., Ph.D.
School of Nursing
University of Washington
Seattle, Washington 98195

T. Berry Brazelton, M.D.
Child Development Unit
Children's Hospital Medical Center
300 Longwood Avenue
Boston, Massachusetts 02115

Jennifer S. Buchwald, Ph.D.
Physiology Department
UCLA School of Medicine
Center for Health Sciences
Los Angeles, California 90024

Cynthia Garcia Coll, Ph.D.
Department of Pediatrics
Women and Infants Hospital
50 Maude Street
Providence, Rhode Island 02908

James T. Dettre
Director of Marketing
  Communications
Johnson & Johnson Baby Products
  Company
Grandview Road
Skillman, New Jersey 08558

Tiffany Field, Ph.D.
Department of Pediatrics
University of Miami
School of Medicine
P.O. Box #016820
1601 N.W. 12th Avenue
Miami, Florida 33101

Joy Goldberger, M.S.
Child Life Department
Johns Hopkins Hospital
600 N. Wolfe Street
Baltimore, Maryland 21205

Peter A. Gorski, M.D.
Department of Pediatrics
Evanston Hospital
2650 Ridge Avenue
Evanston, Illinois 60201

Nina Gunzenhauser
Science Writer
P.O. Box 111
Franklin, New York 13775

Frances Degen Horowitz, Ph.D.
Department of Human Development
University of Kansas
Lawrence, Kansas 66045

Robert L. Isaacson, Ph.D.
Department of Psychology
State University of New York
University Center at Binghamton
Binghamton, New York 13901

Anneliese F. Korner, Ph.D.
Division of Child Psychiatry and
  Child Development
Stanford University Medical Center
San Francisco, California 94305

Barry M. Lester, Ph.D.
Bradley Hospital
1011 Veterans Memorial Parkway
East Providence, Rhode Island 02915

John C. Masters, Ph.D.
Director for Center of Studies of
  Family & Children
Professor of Psychology
Vanderbilt Institute for
  Public Policy Studies
1218 Eighteenth Avenue South
Nashville, Tennessee 37212

Barry Nurcombe, M.D., F.R.A.C.P.
Clinical Director
Bradley Hospital
1011 Veterans Memorial Parkway
East Providence, Rhode Island 02915

Arthur H. Parmelee, M.D.
Department of Pediatrics
UCLA School of Medicine
Los Angeles, California 90024

Bonnie J. Petrauskas
Marketing Communications
    Assistant
Johnson & Johnson Baby Products
    Company
Grandview Road
Skillman, New Jersey 08558

Craig T. Ramey, Ph.D.
Director of Research
Frank Porter Graham Child
    Development Center
Highway 54 Bypass, Building 071A
Chapel Hill, North Carolina 27514

Robert B. Rock, Jr., M.A., M.P.A.
Director of Professional Relations
Johnson & Johnson Baby Products
    Company
Grandview Road
Skillman, New Jersey 08558

Michael L. Schwartz, Ph.D.
Section of Neuroanatomy
Yale University School of Medicine
333 Cedar Street, C-303 SHM
New Haven, Connecticut 06510

D. Nico Spinelli, M.D.
Department of Psychology
University of Massachusetts
    at Amherst
Amherst, Massachusetts 01003

Edward Tronick, Ph.D.
Department of Psychology
University of Massachusetts
    at Amherst
Amherst, Massachusetts 01003

Peter M. Vietze, Ph.D.
Institute for Basic Research in Mental
    Retardation and Developmental
    Disabilities
1050 Forest Hill Road
Staten Island, New York 10314

Doris Welcher, Ph.D.
Behavioral Scientist
The Child Growth and Development
    Corporation
201 West Madison Street
Baltimore, Maryland 21201

Preface

Pediatric Round Table #13 on Infant Stimulation can be viewed as rounding out a "baker's dozen" of Johnson & Johnson Baby Products Company-sponsored programs focusing on the health and development of infants and young children. Under the leadership of an outstanding group of moderators, this series of Round Tables has been made up of multidisciplinary faculties whose members have both national and international reputations and have made significant contributions to the literature in their specialty areas.

As the series, with its broad range of subjects directed primarily to the needs of children in the zero-to-three age bracket, has progressed over the past thirteen years, its audience has expanded to well over half a million health care professionals. More recently, the Round Tables have stimulated consumer publication counterparts, such as TOUCH, The Language of Love, aimed at providing professionals with patient aids. More importantly, they have sought to concentrate on development of Round Table Guidelines. This was a major goal of this latest Round Table.

The planning for Pediatric Round Table #13 began almost two years ago. Its stated program objective was "to review the most recent research information and ideas in the field of infant stimulation, considering both pre- and normal-term infants from the viewpoints of brain plasticity, appropriate levels of stimulation, development and assessment, and intervention, with the ultimate objective of developing guidelines for the recommended policies and procedures to be implemented for the improvement of the quality of patient care." We believe the readers of this publication should be favorably impressed by the manner in which this objective has been pursued.

The Round Table's participants represent a faculty of eighteen experts from the fields of child development, pediatrics, physiology, animal behavior, and neurology. Their specific contributions, the related wide-ranging discussions that followed, and the resulting set of guidelines reflect Round Table consensus and provide a solid basis for theoretical and clinical insights for practical implementation. We hope that child health care professionals concerned with this field will share our feeling of pride in making this state-of-the-art information broadly available.

Robert B. Rock, Jr., M.A., M.P.A.
Director of Professional Relations

INTRODUCTION

The history of this Round Table goes back to a conversation several years ago. We were talking about our experiences over the years in working with preterm infants and about some of the work that was going on in the field, especially about what we knew and didn't know about development in preterm infants and the effects of stimulation on their development. As we talked we became increasingly concerned about how little we understood the mechanisms by which preterm infants react to the environment. We discussed the meaning of behavioral assessments of the preterm and the implications of behavioral assessments for the early detection of the infant at risk for adverse developmental outcome, but we realized that we had no answers. We had questions too about stimulation: what is appropriate stimulation, and what are the potential dangers of stimulation and the ways in which some of the notions of brain plasticity are being used to justify assessment and intervention procedures with preterm infants?

We concluded that it was time for a critical evaluation of these issues, to look at what we do know about brain plasticity and the effects of stimulation and to look at some of the mechanisms of behavioral development and behavioral assessment. We were certain of a few things: that a Johnson & Johnson Round Table would be the ideal forum to bring together the experts, that we wanted the Round Table to have the goal of developing guidelines for infant stimulation, and that we wanted it to produce a statement of recommended policies and procedures for public dissemination. And we knew we wanted each of you here. This Round Table is something of a departure from most previous Round Tables with its mandate for policy recommendations, and we're pleased that Johnson & Johnson took up the challenge.

Barry M. Lester, Ph.D.,
and Edward Tronick, Ph.D.

PROLOGUE

To put our discussion in perspective, we might begin by taking a look at a high-risk special care nursery that would probably look rather strange to all of us. By considering how this care system works, we may bring into focus the issues we will be raising and the terminology we will be using.

The setting is the altiplano of Peru, 13,500 feet above sea level. It is a high-risk situation for the neonate. First, as you know, oxygen level goes down in relationship to altitude. Moreover, exposure to solar radiation is very high at this altitude. Diurnal temperature variations are extremely wide. Typically there are freezing temperatures every night of the year, and as we know from physiologic studies in our intensive care nurseries, as temperature is lowered, there is a very large and rapid increase in the oxygen demands of the infant. Finally, the humidity at this altitude is extremely low. Each of these factors is a form of stress for the infant, and in combination they produce a very high level of risk.

Another risk factor is the size of the infant. Infants at high altitude are born at lower birthweight than are their sea-level cousins. There is a reciprocal relationship between the size of the infant and the size of the placenta, and at high altitudes placental weight tends to be greater than at low altitudes, possibly as an adaptation to maintain the oxygen supply to the fetus. Its cost is the increased risk associated with lower birthweight.

With a somewhat limited technology, the Peruvians have created a special care nursery for their infants to help them survive initially and become acclimatized to this environment. The infant is first completely and very tightly swaddled, with the arms down at the sides, and then dressed in a number of garments made of wool and alpaca. At this stage you can pick a baby up at its center of balance as if it were on a cradle board. In the final step of swaddling, a band about four inches wide is wrapped around the baby, so that only the face is visible.

The infant is then further enclosed in a large blanket, with his head covered, and placed on the mother's back. The wrappings weigh as much as the baby, three to four kilograms, and their thickness is about ten centimeters. The infant has no light stimulation and little auditory stimulation and does not share the mother's temperature regulatory system, because the insulation is far too great.

How does this special care nursery work? Inside the pouch, temperature is maintained at 91 to 93 degrees Fahrenheit. Over short periods of time, that temperature can be maintained whether the pouch is in the sun, where daytime temperatures are 90 to 120 degrees, or in the shade, where daytime temperatures often drop to 40 degrees. The humidity, which in the external environment is about 18 percent relative humidity, is raised inside the pouch to about 50 percent, and the CO_2 content inside the pouch goes up about 20 percent from the ambient environment.

The spaced feeding of these infants occurs at long intervals, in a very perfunctory manner. There is little or no interaction with the infant. The infant is carried on the mother's back, at first with the head slightly lower than the feet. The infant is not changed very often, and there is no specific diaper, just cloths or wraps that help humidify this environment.

All this works together as a caretaking strategy aimed at conserving energy and maximizing growth. States of sleep, probably state 1 sleep, are induced by wrapping the infant, raising the temperature and CO_2 level, supplying movement stimulation through the mother's walking, and by not handling or playing with the infant and limiting other stimulation. Thus demands on the infant's energy are reduced, and more energy can be put into growth. In fact this environment may even induce torpor in these infants, a physiologic state of even lower metabolic rate.

Over the first six months of life, this procedure is modified radically. The infant goes from being tilted down to being put into a vertical position and is gradually unwrapped and exposed to temperature, light, sounds, and the visual environment. We know there is an increase in vital capacity in these infants over time. We think there may be a prolongation of the life of fetal blood, which binds oxygen somewhat better. There is an increased growth velocity for brown fat in these infants, without an increase in linear growth. And motor development is slowed down. Thinking about this special care nursery, we can address a number of issues in terms that we've all been using:

- Is it an environment of maintenance? Is it an environment that facilitates development? Does it induce certain forms of development? Does it indeed enrich development?

- What is the target of this caretaking system? Is it a physiologic system? Is it a motor system? Is it a behavioral state system?

- What effects does this caretaking system have on the brain's development, given the limitation on perceptual input? Is its effect peripheral or central? Does it provide the kind of stimulation that is appropriate for normal brain development?

- How is the timing of this stimulation adjusted? Is it based on a set schedule independent of individual characteristics of the infant, or is it specifically fitted to developmental markers as the infant develops and becomes acclimatized?

- What are the long-term effects of this system? What are the short-term effects?

If we see this as a system functioning to acclimatize these children, with specifically fitted kinds of stimulation and practices modified in terms of timing and quantity, we can ask the two questions that are related most centrally to this conference:

First, how can environments be characterized with respect to their influence on developmental outcomes of the neonate? And second, to what degree should caregivers modify their care to fit the requirements of the individual infant?

Edward Tronick, Ph.D.

PART I
BRAIN
PLASTICITY

A COMPARISON OF PLASTICITY IN SENSORY AND COGNITIVE PROCESSING SYSTEMS

Jennifer S. Buchwald, Ph.D.

For purposes of this Round Table, a working definition of brain plasticity is suggested as "the structural-functional changes produced by endogenous and/or exogenous influences that may occur at any time during the individual's life history." This paper discusses plasticity across species and across brain systems within a species in relation to the central processing of auditory information.

In humans, two electrophysiological measures, the auditory brainstem responses (ABRs) and the cognitive "P300" event-related potential, reflect major developmental differences in the maturation of their brain generator systems. The ABRs, which are generated by the primary auditory pathway of the brainstem, show mature latencies and waveforms by one to two years of age. The P300, which is probably generated by several interacting forebrain systems, does not show a mature configuration until sixteen to eighteen years of age. We hypothesize that such a slowly developing cognitive system will show relatively more plasticity than the more rapidly developing sensory system.

Categories of Brain Plasticity

Under the broad definition given above, there are a number of different categories of brain plasticity: (1) plasticity of the developing brain, with neurogenesis, morphogenesis, synaptogenesis all serving to change the structure and function of component parts and thereby the whole; (2) plasticity of the aging brain, also with changes in structure and function of component parts which in turn reflect upon the whole; (3) plasticity of the acutely lesioned or traumatized brain, with functional recovery intimately related to structural reorganization; and (4) plasticity of the learning brain, with functional, and probably structural, change related to the experience of stimuli that have newly acquired significance.

Within these categories, what does plasticity mean?

The plasticity of development, for example, has been shown to be neither a linear nor a unimodal process. Even for the development of such a simple system as the neuromuscular junction, there is a transient period of superfluous innervation followed by withdrawal of many functional synaptic connections. In the frog, the process of synapse elimination occurs predominantly in the first two to four weeks after metamorphosis, although some remaining polyneuronal innervation is only gradually removed throughout the life of the frog (Morrison- Graham, 1983). Similarly, in the developing rat, there is a progressive loss of polyneuronal innervation of the soleus muscle which results in a reduction of motor unit size to the adult pattern (Brown, Jansen, & Van Essen, 1976). Although development is generally characterized by proliferation, by more growth, more differentiation, more functional contacts, these data emphasize that it is difficult to second-guess nature: more is not necessarily better or even the norm.

Many different forms of plasticity are under the control of a variety of mechanisms that are only beginning to be understood. For example, cortical neurons of kittens show accelerated postnatal expansion of their dendritic fields; concurrently, neurons in the brainstem reticular formation progressively shrink during development (Scheibel & Scheibel, 1958). Still a third pattern of development is exemplified by some of the sensory relay neurons, which are structurally and functionally adult-like at birth and show relatively little postnatal change (Pujol & Hilding, 1973).

During aging, the brain may exhibit plastic changes that are also characteristic of development. Brain areas with significant cell loss due to aging may contain surviving cells with dendritic arborizations that have expanded into adjacent denervated territory (Scheibel & Tomiyasu, 1978). An extreme example of adult brain plasticity has recently been demonstrated in the canary, in which neurogenesis, previously thought to terminate at birth, continues to occur and establish functional circuitry in the brain throughout adulthood (Paton & Nottebohm, 1984).

Electrophysiological Probes of Brain Function

Surface-recorded electrophysiological responses have the tremendous advantage of being simple, noninvasive probes of brain function that can be used repeatedly on any one individual for longitudinal studies of development or on different age groups for horizontal norms of development. For a number of years in my laboratory we have been studying the central processing of auditory information, in part as revealed by scalp-recorded evoked potentials in human subjects and in the cat as an experimental model (reviewed in Buchwald, 1982; in press). An evoked potential is the brain wave response produced by the presentation of a particular stimulus, such as a click or a tone. In both human and cat, these potentials commence with a latency of one or two milliseconds after stimulus onset and extend through time for 500 milliseconds or more. (Latency is the time of occurrence after stimulus onset.) If the primary generator substrate of a particular evoked potential component can be defined, that component then becomes a convenient analytical electrophysiological probe. Thus, changes in the latency, amplitude, or general morphology of a particular auditory evoked response component can be used to assess the functioning of its generator substrate system during early development as well as during the protracted changes of old age, during acute trauma and chronic disease, or simply during physiological challenges imposed by parametric manipulations of the stimulus.

The development of two human evoked potential components will be contrasted in this discussion: the short-latency auditory brainstem response and the long-latency cognitive P300 response.

Development of auditory function: The "ABR" index. The auditory brainstem responses (ABRs) represent a significant watershed in the recent history of human scalp-recorded evoked potentials. This sequence of five evoked potential components occurs in response to click stimuli within a very short latency range of 1 to 10 milliseconds.

The waveform of each ABR component is short in duration (about 1 millisecond) and does not change, even when clicks are presented as rapidly as ten or twenty per second (indicating a rapid recovery cycle). During the 1970s, a major international effort was undertaken to determine the origin of these short-latency potentials through animal experiments designed to provide specific pieces of information. Moreover, for the first time, potentials with similar electrophysiological characteristics—that is, the ABRs—were demonstrated to be present in animal models and in the human and to have similar neural substrates, the auditory brainstem pathway. And for the first time, there was international consensus on this aspect of the human scalp-recorded evoked potential sequence. As a result, ABRs are now widely used in humans to screen for possible impairment of sound transmission within the auditory pathway and as a more general electrophysiological measure of brainstem function.

ABRs have been used extensively in neonatal and premature nurseries to evaluate ABR waveform, latency, and recovery cycle characteristics for both normal infants and those whose hearing or brainstem viability is at risk. A great advantage of this measure is that it is not influenced by changes in attention or arousal levels. The large normative data base that has been collected over the past ten years indicates that while the anatomy of the peripheral and caudal brainstem of the human auditory system is relatively mature at birth (Hecox, 1975), functional development continues through the first year or two of life. In a study of full-term newborns and infants six weeks, three months, six months, and one year of age, as well as of normal adults, the adult waveform configuration was found to replace the infantile response by three to six months (Salamy & McKean, 1976). Peripheral transmission, reflected by ABR wave 1, reached adult latency by the sixth week, while central transmission time through the brainstem (waves 1-5) matured more slowly and did not match that of the adult until approximately one year (Salamy & McKean, 1976). Recovery cycles to click rates ranging from ten to forty per second were functionally mature at birth for peripheral and caudal brainstem structures (waves 1-3), whereas recovery cycles of waves generated by more rostral brainstem structures (waves 4, 5) were not mature for several weeks postnatally (Salamy et al., 1978). These findings are consistent with the general finding of a caudo-rostral progression of neurodevelopment, and with the extensively studied structural-functional development of the auditory system in the kitten (Pujol & Hilding, 1973; Buchwald & Shipley, in press).

Studies of premature infants indicate that reliable ABR

components first appear at about the 28th week of gestation, although with relatively loud stimuli unstable ABRs can be recorded somewhat earlier (Starr et al., 1977; Krumholz et al., 1985). Complementary behavioral data indicate that blink-startle responses to vibroacoustic stimulation, monitored ultrasonically in human fetuses, are first elicited between 24 and 25 weeks of gestational age and are consistently present after 28 weeks (Birnholz & Benacerraf, 1983). The waveform variability and latencies of the ABR components decrease rapidly as gestation proceeds, with a maximal rate of change between 28 and 34 weeks (Starr et al., 1977; Krumholz et al., 1985). In an important comparison study, longitudinal postnatal recordings from preterm infants (30-35 weeks' gestation) were found to show the same ABR waveform and latency as those of infants born at later gestational ages (Starr et al., 1977; Krumholz et al., 1985).

Taken together, these studies indicate that the ABRs provide an objective means for quantifying functional development of the auditory system in the human infant, independent of factors of arousal or attention, and for assessing the effects of environmental and congenital factors during the critical period after birth. Longitudinal recordings of preterm infants and comparisons with infants born at later gestational ages have led to the conclusion that maturation of auditory function proceeds at about the same rate in extrauterine and intrauterine environments.

Development of cognitive function: The P300 index. The P300 response is a scalp-recorded, computer-averaged evoked potential that appears in the human subject as a large positive voltage in the 300 to 500 millisecond latency range and reflects a variety of cognitive brain functions. In contrast to the ABRs, the P300 is relatively independent of the physical characteristics of the evoking stimulus but is very sensitive to endogenous variables and to task requirements related to the stimulus. The P300 response has been intensively studied over the past decade. It is elicited by rare or omitted stimuli that occur randomly in a series of expected stimuli, and it appears to be a neural correlate of such cognitive functions as sequential information processing, short-term memory, and/or decision-making (Squires et al., 1976, 1977; Ford et al., 1980; Donchin, 1981).

The P300 has become increasingly interesting to neurologists, psychiatrists, and other clinicians insofar as it is missing or abnormal in some kinds of brain disease, such as Alzheimer's disease and schizophrenia. In normal aging, without associated disease, the P300 progressively increases in latency and diminishes in amplitude, but with significantly less change than that observed in age-matched demented subjects (Goodin, Squires, & Starr, 1978; Pfefferbaum et al., 1980; Syndulko et al., 1982; Picton et al., 1984). Thus, the P300 reflects a change in cognitive brain function associated with age but reflects relatively more intense changes as a function of particular brain diseases.

Relatively little is known about the developmental history of the P300. While long-latency event-related potentials have been recorded from infants as young as six months, P300 responses have not been clearly identified in children younger than six to eight years (Courchesne, 1979). Whether or not P300 waves may be found in infants and younger children awaits future research. By six to eight years, however, the P300 appears as a large amplitude, long-duration positivity that peaks at a latency of about 700 milliseconds; by ten to thirteen years the P300 latency is still prolonged at 600 milliseconds, and its amplitude and waveform are still immature. Gradually, during the period of development ranging from fourteen to seventeen years, the P300 waveform and latency acquire adult values (Courchesne, 1979).

In our own P300 research, we are pursuing studies of linguistic and prosodic processing in children and adults, and in normal and clinical populations. Prosody, the intonational component of language that conveys emotional state such as anger or happiness, has, for example, been reported to be absent from the speech of higher-functioning autistic children who can produce linguistically appropriate sentences.

We have used the following stimuli in typical rare/frequent configurations for P300 studies of several different subject groups:

Phoneme pairs: ba/pa
Word pairs: rip/lip
Prosodic (linguistic) pairs: Bob (statement)/Bob (question)
Prosodic (affective) pairs: Bob (angry)/Bob (happy)

In general, the P300 responses that showed the longest latencies were those to the "rip"/"lip" word pair. These results are consistent with the general finding that P300 latencies increase as discrimination becomes more difficult and suggest that different or additional brain systems must be engaged as the task requirements become more difficult.

In a study designed to assess functional plasticity of cognitive development, we compared responses recorded from a group of adults with

English as a first language with responses from a group of adults with Japanese as a first language (but fluent in both speaking and writing English). The two groups showed essentially the same P300 responses to the phonemic and prosodic stimulus pairs. However, the word pair "rip"/"lip," which produced clear P300 responses in the English language group, evoked essentially no P300 response in the Japanese language group. These results indicate that at some cognitive level the brain of the Japanese language subjects is unable to discriminate the "r" and "l" sounds.

Supportive behavioral data were obtained from an additional test in which the subjects were presented with twenty balanced pairs of "r"/"l" words in a two-choice, forced-choice design. For example, when the word "rock" was played from the stimulus tape, the subject had to circle either "rock" or "lock" on the answer sheet. English first-language speakers scored 100 percent on this test, while many of the Japanese scored at chance levels, and as a group the Japanese scored significantly lower than the English speakers.

These results suggest that the acoustic—that is, linguistic— environment during development is responsible for developmental differences in the brain. There is a diminished or absent capacity at the cognitive level of the P300, but not at the input level of the ABRs, to discriminate certain complex sounds not included in the phonology of the native language.

Differential Functional Plasticity of the Developing Brain

The ABR and P300 responses serve to illustrate dramatic differences in the functional development of the sensory and cognitive processing systems in the human. Clearly, the ABRs are mature at an age—one to two years—when the P300 cannot even be recorded. What does this mean in terms of the functional development of the brain? One of the most conservative interpretations might be that auditory stimuli are gaining ready access to the brain almost from birth, but the brain only very gradually, very slowly, begins to be able to use and to process those stimuli in a cognitive fashion. The long lag in P300 development strongly indicates a biological immaturity in those cognitive brain systems necessary for sequential information processing and recent memory functions. However, the inability of adults to discriminate P300 stimuli not in the phonology of their native language indicates that at some point the P300 system becomes nonplastic and biased away from stimuli not heard during development.

DISCUSSION

Arthur Parmelee: Quite a few of us have been interested in comparing neurophysiological development in preterm infants and in kittens. In many ways the neurophysiological development of the kitten in the first three weeks of life is like that of the preterm infant. It is my impression that the decibel level has to be quite high to induce brainstem evoked potentials and that the frequency range is narrower in the kitten in the first weeks of life compared with the kitten of three weeks of age. The point is that early on there may in fact be a peripheral sensory protective mechanism.

Jennifer Buchwald: I think that in the Starr et al. paper, as well as in our own studies with the kitten, that point is made—that the intensity of the stimulus necessary to induce the potential has to be greater. But if the intensity is increased in the kitten, then the response can be induced. The increased threshold appears to be very largely due to mechanical factors in the middle ear.

Arthur Parmelee: Also, I think Pujol demonstrated that in the very young kitten the response to the stimulus was only to the onset of the sound and that there was an inability to follow duration of the sound stimulus. Thus, a response could be obtained unrelated to the information in the stimulus, because whatever went on after the initial onset of the signal wasn't followed by neuronal responses. The fact that you can get a reaction—either evoked potential or a body movement— early in preterm life doesn't mean that you are getting a lot of information in.

Jennifer Buchwald: What about the responses of very young infants to mothers' voices, for instance? Has anybody looked at that in preterm infants?

Arthur Parmelee: Essentially not below 35 or 36 weeks conceptional age.

Jennifer Buchwald: It might be that there is a considerable difference. On the other hand, I think it was a surprise to most people that term infants, or infants very soon after birth, showed so much auditory discrimination to voices.

Nico Spinelli: I have difficulty with the P300. P300, I was told, means a positivity at 300 milliseconds after the stimulus. But then all the workers on P300 are happy to tell you whether a certain P300 has a latency of 500 milliseconds or 400. How is that possible?

Jennifer Buchwald: I can't really tell you how it got to be named. I think it reflects a process more than a potential. In the example I showed you from our own data, where the same kinds of stimuli are presented, in the "rip"/"lip" situation the discrimination is more difficult, and we get a P300 potential shifted in latency. This suggests that more or different brain systems are being engaged, or they are having to work harder, or they are having to work through more sequences of operations in order to get that discrimination made.

Robert Isaacson: But if I understand Nico, I think he was asking why it couldn't be that early in life you get a P700 and then at some later time a P300 develops. There may or may not be a gradual change.

Nico Spinelli: Not only that, but I'm actually suggesting something more radical: Given that we do have a so-called P300 to an auditory task, or to a linguistic task, or to a visual task, we can evoke a P300 every time there is something either infrequent or amiss or surprising in a variety of cognitive tasks taking place in completely different systems. But all we are really seeing is one system—let's say vision—saying, hey, there is something unusual going on here. Now, vision would take a time different from audition, and that would tell us not that we have many different delays in the same process but that the same process is performed by different systems. Could that be possible?

Jennifer Buchwald: Actually, most of the work on the P300 has been done with visual stimuli. There is an increased latency in the primary visual system, so that a visual cortical potential occurs at 25 or 30 milliseconds and an auditory cortical occurs at 12 to 15 milliseconds. But that latency difference is relatively small compared with the latency of the so-called P300 potential, so that with either visual stimuli or auditory stimuli it occurs at about the same time. We think of this response as due to a series of interacting systems that are processing information, and the difference in the latency of the sensory response per se doesn't seem to be important. We're still at a very crude level in evaluating all this, but the difficulty of discrimination seems to make the most difference, rather than the stimulus modality.

Edward Tronick: Have you done any phonetic training with the Japanese to see if you can get a P300?

Jennifer Buchwald: No, we have not, but we do have a smaller group of about six subjects who grew up in Japan and who have lived in the United States for up to fifteen years. One cannot do this discrimination at all, even though he has been speaking English for fifteen years. On the other hand, some of those who have just come from Japan are able to do the discrimination even a month later. Overall, as a group, it doesn't seem to make any difference whether they are in the United States for a long period or not.

Berry Brazelton: Do you have any babies that were born over here that you have compared with babies born in Japan?

Jennifer Buchwald: No, but my colleague, Dr. Kaga, who inspired this study, has a large population in Japan and we are going to do this same study over there.

Berry Brazelton: If they were bilingual from the first, would they have the discrimination?

Jennifer Buchwald: We haven't looked at that, but I am sure that if they were bilingual they would have the "rip"/"lip" discrimination.

BRAIN PLASTICITY AFTER DAMAGE

Robert L. Isaacson, Ph.D.

In my laboratory we are motivated by three goals: (1) learning how to prevent brain damage, (2) learning how to reduce the anatomical and pathophysiological consequences of brain damage, and (3) learning how to reduce the mental and behavioral effects of brain damage.

We are interested in trying to reach these goals in individuals of all ages, not only in the young and not only in the elderly. The quality of life is important at all ages.

The Prevention of Brain Damage

We are just beginning to appreciate the significance of environmental pollutants and toxins, not to mention "individually programmed" pharmacologic interventions (street drugs), on the development of the individual. Some recent examples of the devastation that have been seen to be produced by such means, thalidomide aside, may be the fetal alcohol syndrome and the chemically instigated instances of Parkinson's disease induced by the street drug MTPT. Just as we are finding that many cancers can be traced back to the incorporation of some toxin or some other form of environmental contaminant, so we will find that some mental aberrancies have a similar origin. If a particular toxin does not itself produce abnormalities, its secondary effects through the cardiovascular, hepatic, or immune systems may.

The effects of sodium nitrite on the brain and on behavior have had increasing interest to me. Sodium nitrite is commonly added to foods to prevent formation of *botulinum* toxin. The use of nitrites has come under greater criticism than the use of nitrates because they are chemically more easily converted to nitrosamine, agents with established carcinogenic properties. However, my concern has been with the effect of the nitrite as it converts the iron of the heme molecule from the ferrous (Fe^{2+}) to the ferric state (Fe^{3+}), producing methemoglobin at the expense of hemoglobin. Since methemoglobin cannot be used to provide oxygen to bodily tissues, a hypoxic state results.

The acute administration of sodium nitrite produces a hypoxic condition in rats. We have used doses between 50 and 100 mg/kg, most often 75 mg/kg, which produces a very noticeable short-term effect in the hippocampal formation. Most of our studies have used rats given a single large dose of the nitrite and sacrificed 24 hours later, although we have found similar effects after chronic administration of lower doses. Despite the obvious "distressed" nature of many cells in the hippocampus of animals sacrificed 24 hours after the nitrite, this effect is not permanent, or not obviously so, and if several days are allowed to elapse between the nitrite administration and sacrifice, many fewer cells with abnormal characteristics, and sometimes none at all, are found. Careful metabolic and membrane studies need to be done on the cells as they recover from nitrite administration.

In pilot studies now underway, we have preliminary evidence that the pretreatment of rats with 5.0 mg/kg of nimodipine, a calcium slow channel antagonist, can prevent the usual cellular deterioration produced by the nitrites. The drug seems to provide protection for the cells in the areas most frequently damaged by the nitrite, that is, the hippocampus and the neocortical surface.

In other studies, we have evaluated the percentage of methemoglobin produced by our chronic injections. In one study it was found that the stress of a single injection of a small amount of physiological saline two hours or even 24 hours before the nitrite administration produced a profound reduction in the methemoglobin formed by the nitrite—about 30 to 40 percent—relative to the amount found in untreated animals (Fahey, 1986).

Conversely, we have some recent data that suggest that the effect of the nitrites on behavior and methemoglobin formation is greatly enhanced by the pretreatment with drugs characteristic of a major tranquilizer. This suggests to me that while a low level of nitrite incorporation may not be dangerous to the normal, vigorous, somewhat stressed child, a child or infant that is quiet, perhaps because of a tranquilizer or certain antiseizure medications, may be in much greater jeopardy.

Originally we thought that the doses we gave were well beyond any physiological levels that would be found in people. However, evaluation of commercially available hot dogs, which usually contain 200-250 mg of sodium nitrite per hot dog, turned up one brand, kept in the frozen food section of a local supermarket and labeled "no preservatives or nitrites added," that contained 1,500 mg per hot dog. Three or four of these hot dogs would deliver a nitrite dose in the same range we have been studying. Even accepting the lower levels found in most hot dogs, it is an open question as to how much total nitrite people really take in each day through their drinking water and other foods such as bologna, chicken breasts, and canned meats and what the chronic effects of these amounts are.

The Reduction of Brain Damage

A second, related area of research that has engaged my interest is the reduction of brain damage induced by ischemia or hypoxia produced by cardiac abnormalities or by stroke.

We are just beginning to understand that the brain, as well as a number of other organs, can withstand substantial periods of oxygen deprivation. Brain tissues can recover essentially normal physiological characteristics after thirty minutes of oxygen deprivation; the liver may be able to withstand three hours of such privation.

The real killer of cells subjected to oxygen deprivation is the activation of certain excitatory amino acid receptors, when oxygen is again available to the cells (see, for example, Wieloch, 1985). The activation of these receptors in turn opens calcium channels and also causes the release of intracellular calcium stores. The net effect is to destroy permanently the energy-producing capabilities of the mitochondria, producing cell death.

The amount of tissue damage resulting from global or regional ischemia can be greatly reduced by elimination of calcium from the immediate environment of the cell or by the blockade of the calcium slow channels by appropriate pharmacologic agents. In my laboratory we have been primarily interested in the effects of one of these calcium slow channel blocking agents, nimodipine, a drug that has special effectiveness in brain blood vessels and tissues (Fleckenstein, 1981; Heistad & Haws, 1985). An important question is whether or not administration of this drug can reduce the anatomical or physiological consequences of brain damage. At least in the cardiovascular system, it is clear that the earlier the drug treatment after the insult, the better the outcome (Scriabine et al., 1985) and that the best protective effects are found when the animals are given the drug prior to an insult, including the induction of hypoxia (Kazda & Hoffmeister, 1979; Hoffmeister et al., 1982).

In some preliminary studies, Bartkowsky and his associates in San Francisco have found that the pretreatment of rats with nimodipine greatly reduces the amount of brain tissue that shows reduced metabolic activity following electrocoagulation of the middle cerebral artery. We have undertaken similar studies using rats in which this artery was ligated. We also studied the animals over a much longer recovery time. The use of the nitro-BT metabolic stain revealed only small differences between the nimodipine-treated and the vehicle-injected animals. However, one study suggests that the long-term beneficial effects of nimodipine treatment will be found to a greater extent in animals with damage restricted to the neocortex than in animals with subcortical involvement (Hardy, 1985).

Reducing the Mental and Behavioral Effects of Brain Damage

Probably our most extensive work over the past several years has involved attempts to compensate animals for the loss of hippocampal tissue. Our basic approach is to create large bilateral hippocampal lesions by aspiration and then to study the changes that usually follow the damage. We have chosen this lesion model for a very simple re᠎ ᠎n: we know the distribution of effects that follow such lesions (see, for example, Isaacson, 1982).

In using the term *distribution of effects,* I want to emphasize that apparently identical lesions, whether made in adulthood or in infancy, can produce a variety of consequences, depending in part on genetic and experimental factors (Donovick & Burright, 1984) and in part on idiopathic variables. For example, György Buzsaki and I recently studied the level of hyperactivity of fifty rats with hippocampal damage as compared with a like number of animals with damage to the neocortex alone or animals subjected to sham operations. As a group the animals with hippocampal damage were unquestionably more active than those in the other two groups, but within that group there was a wide range of activity scores. The scores obtained by a particular animal do not depend on the size or location of the lesion of the hippocampus. Furthermore, with repeated testing, an animal's score on one day is not a good predictor of its score on the next.

One of my basic assumptions for research using various specific and general intervention procedures is that if one could restore remaining neural systems to something like their status before (or without) the damage, behaviors mediated by those systems could be "normalized," at least to some degree. Our intervention studies first targeted the forebrain dopaminergic systems. We were most interested in understanding the significance of the pathways that connect the ventral subiculum of the hippocampal formation to the ventromedial portions of the caudate and to nucleus accombens. There was strong biochemical evidence (Springer & Isaacson, 1982) that after hippocampal lesions, the release and metabolism of dopamine in these regions was reduced. Therefore, we undertook to simulate an enhancement of dopamine release in these basal ganglia regions by the direct injection of a dopamine agonist into these regions. We used a direct micro-injection of DPI (3,4-dihydroxyphenyl-amino-2-imidazoline), a dopamine agonist for the mesolimbic dopamine system, which eliminated almost entirely the hyperactivity induced by bilateral destruction of the hippocampus (Reinstein, Hannigan, & Isaacson, 1982).

However, despite our success with the direct dopamine intervention procedures, we realized that this technique offered little promise as a potential application to the human. Therefore we undertook two systemic pharmacologic approaches directed at remedying the hyperactivity produced by bilateral hippocampal destruction: (1) the systemic administration of choline, and (2) the elimination or reduction of endogenous corticosteroids.

Choline, given peripherally, produces alterations in brain "free choline" and acetylcholine levels that exhibit both temporal and regional differences after administration (Wecker, Dettbarn, & Schmidt, 1978; Wecker & Dettbarn, 1979). These changes are found only after procedures that produce a reduction in the animals' normal cholinergic activity levels. It can be argued that hippocampal damage effectively reduces cholinergic effects, because the lesioned animals have an exaggerated sensitivity to the administration of muscarinic blockers.

In a series of studies (Springer, Ryan, & Isaacson, unpublished; Isaacson, Springer, & Ryan, 1986), 100 mg/kg of free base choline, given peripherally, was found to produce a strong but transient reduction in the hyperactivity of the lesioned animals. This effect does not last very long and corresponds to the time at which "free choline" levels are highest in the basal ganglia. Because this "window of normalcy" produced by the systemic choline is so brief, this approach is limited in its practical application. At present we do not know appropriate methods to deliver the choline or other cholinergic agonists to the brain for a long enough time to allow an extended period of "normalized" behavior.

In 1976 Iuvone and Van Hartesveldt found that surgical adrenalectomy radically reduced the hyperactivity often found after bilateral hippocampal lesions. As often happens with results that do not fit in with what is scientifically popular at the time, the paper was repressed by the collective academic mind. However, in 1983, Nyakas, De Kloet, Veldhuis, and Bohus reported a similar result in animals with kainic acid lesions of the hippocampus. About that time, quite independently, we undertook the study of the effects of chemical adrenalectomy on the behavior of animals with hippocampal lesions. We used the drug metyrapone, which interferes with corticosterone synthesis. The effects of the drug are rapid and profound: a 90 percent reduction of the corticosteroids within ten minutes has been reported. The effect of the drug lasts for several hours. With a dose of 25 mg/kg of metyrapone in a tartaric acid vehicle, animals with hippocampal lesions were restored to essentially normal levels of activity, while the behavior of the control animals was unchanged (Ryan et al., 1985).

We recognized that adrenalectomy and metyrapone treatments have a number of effects other than the reduction of the glucocorticoids, and to determine if the behavioral effects were truly the consequence of corticosterone reduction we tried to offset the beneficial effects of metyrapone with supplementation with exogenous hormone. We had only partial success in restoring the hippocampal lesion syndrome by this means, indicating that metyrapone was producing effects in addition to those due to corticosterone depletion. One of these other effects is the induction of an adrenergic supersensitivity. To try to understand the significance of this phenomenon, we induced adrenergic supersensitivity by another means, the administration of bretylium, in animals with hippocampal damage. After the supersensitivity had been produced, we administered low doses of norepinephrine (4 mg/kg) to animals with hippocampal lesions as well as to groups with only cortical damage or to sham operated animals. The norepinephrine failed to influence the lesion-induced hyperactivity. However, despite this failure, norepinephrine restored the hippocampally lesioned animals' ability to exhibit spontaneous alternation.

For reasons yet to be uncovered, these striking results of peripherally administered catecholamines occur only after adrenergic supersensitivity has been induced, although the method used to induce it appears to be immaterial—that is, metyrapone or bretylium. Similar results cannot be obtained by simply increasing the dose of norepinephrine given; a supersensitivity must have been induced beforehand.

It appears, then, that after hippocampal damage a number of alterations occur in known, and sometimes unknown, systems of the brain. Furthermore, it seems clear that we can dissociate various components of the lesion-produced syndrome by the ways in which they can be adjusted or eliminated. This indicates that there will be no "magic bullet" that will make the lesioned animal normal, but we can, at least, take steps toward minimizing one or more of the most devastating effects by appropriate intervention procedures.

At this time, the greatest hope for effective remedial intervention comes from the choline and metyrapone studies. However, I am also reminded of the comments of a psychiatrist some twenty years ago at a conference on mental retardation. He said that the most significant contribution to the elimination of mental retardation in his city would be the elimination of lead-based paints from the walls of ghetto apartments, an intervention second in effectiveness to the elimination of the ghettos themselves. Today, we would have to extend his advice to include the elimination of a host of newly discovered or greatly enhanced toxins and pollutants. The prevention and reduction of brain damage depends on both scientific and environmental-social advances.

DISCUSSION

Nico Spinelli: When you give sodium nitrite to your rats, you say that after stress, the rats withstand the situation better. It should be exactly the opposite, right?

Robert Isaacson: Stress exerts its influence on the amount of methemoglobin produced by the sodium nitrite, not on its anatomic or behavioral consequences. We were amazed that a "blue rat" could easily balance itself on a rotating rod. The blueness of the animals reflects the amount of methemoglobin that has been produced. It's a sign of an effective injection into the animal. However, we could find no *behavioral* effects of this until we first forced the animals to run a bit or to swim for three to five minutes—that is, to engage in some oxygen-consuming enterprise. After such exercise these animals are terrible in tasks requiring motor coordination. When we created a transient oxygen debt through exercise, that's when motoric behavior declined.

Nico Spinelli: I wonder if there might not be a direct toxicity effect from the sodium nitrite itself. I don't know how zinc and sodium nitrite interact, but just as it does something to that iron atom, from one bond state to the other, it could do something to the zinc in the hippocampus. And it is known that if you deplete zinc in the hippocampus you have a hippocampal deficit effect.

Robert Isaacson: Right. However, the zinc distribution doesn't correspond to the distribution of damage caused by the nitrite.

Jennifer Buchwald: Bob, in the manipulation you were doing with the hippocampally lesioned animals, since you could restore the deficits induced by the lesion, what do you think the hippocampus is doing? Do you view it more as a controlling system that can change the balance of activities of this or that system, those using monoamines or cholinergic transmitters, or do you think that the hippocampus is actually responsible for a particular function?

Robert Isaacson: The answer to your last question is no. I don't think any of us, even the youngest person in this room, will live to the point where we understand what the hippocampus does. In regard to the first part of the question, I think you're pretty close to being right. The hippocampus shows its greatest influence on behavior when the environment is uncertain, exactly when your P300 wave shows the greatest increase. I thought that was a wonderful correlation: the two observations fit in so beautifully. I think that when the environment is not as anticipated, then it exerts its influences through a variety of pathways, and one of the pathways is into the basal ganglia, where it alters the dopamine and catecholamine interactions. Now, to me that does not indicate what the hippocampus does, but it is manipulating other systems, especially when the environment is uncertain. And I think that's about all one can say about it.

Michael Schwartz: I'm also curious about what you said about the killing of cells in hypoxia. You suggested that it really wasn't the lack of oxygen but the release of transmitters when function was restored. Does that mean that you believe you could probably go through the brain and map out distributions of various excitatory transmitters and predict which areas might be at risk?

Robert Isaacson: In a way I think that's already been done with people who have suffered cardiac arrest and animals with interrupted blood supplies to their brains. In people, PET scans show regionally reduced metabolic activities for up to three to five years. It would be very interesting to compare those areas with the location of the various excitatory amino acid receptors. On the other hand, the evidence that I think is most convincing comes from experiments with rabbit retina. You can have a rabbit retina suspended in a chamber totally anaerobic for thirty minutes, and if you then reintroduce oxygen without calcium in the medium or with calcium channel blockers, that tissue becomes totally viable again. Others have shown the same sort of thing with liver tissue. I think this approach to cell death is one of the most exciting things that has come along recently.

Nico Spinelli: Some years ago there were some experiments on hypoxia that showed that the dura around the spinal cord can form a compression chamber where you can put a hydrostatic pressure around the spinal cord greater than the blood pressure. You can stop the blood flow without having to close off all the little blood vessels. The blood will actually be squeezed out of the cord. Thus, you don't have problems associated with a blood clot forming. If you do that, you can stop the circulation of the spinal cord for an hour and when you release the pressure everything is working perfectly fine.

Now, why doesn't it work in the head? When I went to medical school, I was taught that the reason the baby's head can linger so long in the birth canal under pressure is that the boney plates of the skull have not sutured and so they can spread apart as needed. As they do so, the head becomes smaller. Now why doesn't the baby pop out brain-damaged every time? It will, of course, if it sits there for too long. The reason it isn't brain-damaged is that when greater blood flow than normal occurs to the brain, the skull can adjust appropriately.

PLASTICITY TRIGGERING EXPERIENCES, NATURE, AND THE DUAL GENESIS OF BRAIN STRUCTURE AND FUNCTION

D. Nico Spinelli, M.D.

The brain responds to experience by adaptively changing its structure, which is initially determined genetically. At no time is this power greater than during critical periods of development. Different experiences, however, do not trigger brain plasticity to the same extent.

We have identified a class of experiences capable of inducing massive changes in the structure and function of visual, somatic, and motor cortex of otherwise normally reared kittens. We refer to these as plasticity triggering experiences (PTEs). We have shown that relatively simple PTEs induce adaptive changes in dendritic trees, dendritic bundles, functional properties of single cells in visual and somato-sensory cortex, and even in the shape of the cortical representation of the body surface and motor map.

These changes are permanent and result in behavioral modifications. PTEs thus seem to influence strongly the direction and extent of future neuro-behavioral activity.

This paper describes research into the creation and effects of PTEs and discusses the implications of this research for the rearing of human infants.

Configuring the Brain

The human brain is an immensely complex structure that has evolved to enable humans to survive and achieve goals in remarkably complex and diverse environments. Mammalian brains in general, and human brains in particular, exhibit powerful adaptive and plastic capabilities. In fact, it is precisely because of these capabilities that the central nervous system can cope with damage, aging, and most importantly with an everchanging environment. It is nothing short of astonishing that humans can cope with a modern world that is almost totally unlike the one that prevailed for hundreds of thousands of years.

The fundamental structure of the brain is determined genetically, but in the last two decades it has become clear that that is only the starting point. The brain as designed and constructed by the genome is not fully configured. Full configuration takes place after birth and is guided by stimuli, information, and challenges that originate in and are specific to a particular environment.

The concept of configuring is borrowed from computer science. It means providing full specification to systems that have to be different in different environments. It means allocating finite resources in ways that are most advantageous for the tasks that lie in the future. Brain systems have to be capable of self-configuration under guidance from the environment, because the environment is unknown until after birth.

Actually the brain has to cope with two environments—the external one and the internal one. The interfaces to the external world must be attuned to *that* world for both the sensory and the motor systems; generalization to all possible worlds would be not only impossible but counterproductive. *Domain specific knowledge* must be built in to make future behavior and successful coping with the environment almost effortless. On the surface it would seem that the interface to the inner world could be determined by the genome, but even here stimuli delivered during development have an impact.

Plasticity Triggering Experiences

Our goal was to explore the effect of visual experience during development on the configuration of visual cortex. For this research we used kittens, whose critical period of configuration lasts just a few weeks after birth. In order to determine that the experience had in fact effected a change in visual cortex, we had to create for the kitten a unique experience, one that would never occur naturally and whose effects we could recognize as such in visual cortex. This seemingly impossible requirement was quite easily achieved by putting goggles on the kitten's eyes so that a danger stimulus could be presented to one eye only. The danger signal required the kitten to lift one of the front legs or receive a mild shock on the forearm. A safe stimulus was presented to the other eye on correct performance. In their evolutionary history cats have never had this experience of seeing different stimuli in the two eyes, so it is unique. On the other hand, the stimuli used (vertical bars for one eye and horizontal bars for the other) are normal, and the situation—dealing successfully with a small danger—is also quite normal for a kitten. The experience was given once a day for eight minutes. The kittens learned it very quickly.

We then studied the functional neuroanatomy of single cells in visual cortex by mapping their receptive fields with the aid of a minicomputer. The computer moves a small disc on a screen which is imaged on the retina of the cat, while simultaneously recording the activity of a single cortical cell via a microelectrode. The computer generates a two-dimensional map of the regions where the disc elicits a response in the cell examined. This is the visual receptive field for that cell.

What we found was that the receptive fields of cells responding to the horizontally stimulated eye were oriented horizontally; those of cells responding to the vertically stimulated eye were vertical. Figure 1 shows such a map of a receptive field. There are three horizontal bars, in an almost iconic reproduction of the experience.

Thus the unique nature of the experience had engendered in visual cortex a population of cells with equally unique response properties. These neurons could be activated by the left or by the right eye, but they were most responsive to vertical bars for one eye and horizontal bars for the other. In animals that have not received this type of experience, stimulus selectivity is the same for both eyes.

Effects on Sensory and Motor Cortex

Our expectations were that the experience described above would not only produce changes in the response properties of cells in visual cortex but would produce modifications of responses in the cells of sensory cortex as well. We owe to Penfield (Penfield & Boldrey, 1937) the finding that on the anterior surface of the cerebral hemisphere the

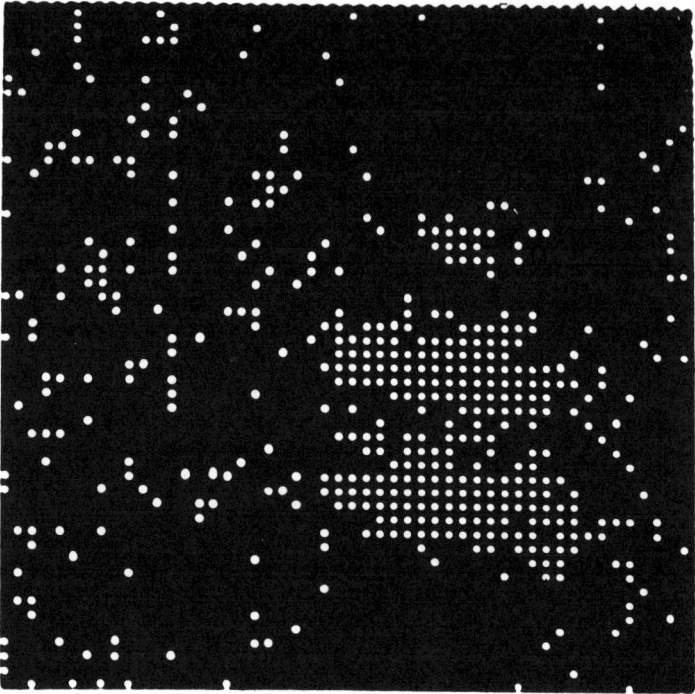

Figure 1.   Map of receptive field of visual cortex cells associated with eye
stimulated by horizontal pattern.

sensory surface of the body is mapped topologically in the "sensory
homunculus" and the motor apparatus is mapped in the "motor
homunculus." Penfield had pointed out that the amount of cortex
occupied by a body part relates not to the size of that part but to its
sensory or motor sophistication. Thus in humans the fingertips
occupy large areas of cortex and the torso only a small one.

Many of the cells in the sensory representation are
polysensory—that is, they respond to more than one sensory
modality—and we were hoping that the area mapping the forearm
involved in the training would respond to the visual stimuli used. In
our kittens we found not only that this was true but that the area
mapping the trained forearm was several times larger than the area
mapping the untrained one. We also found that of the polysensory
cells a very large percentage responded to the danger stimulus, even
though the kittens had observed this stimulus for a total of only a few
minutes. The next highest percentage of polysensory cells responded
to the safe stimulus, which had been observed cumulatively for hours.
Finally there were cells that responded to everyday stimuli, even

though from the point of view of time these had constituted the much larger experience of the kittens. Naturally, there is only so much real estate on the cortical surface, and this enlargement comes at the expense of a compression of nearby representations.

We decided to run another study (Spinelli & Jensen, 1982) to investigate if any changes in the motor representations of our kittens had been produced by the early experience. By now I was convinced that early stimulation was changing the brain interface to the external world and decided that quite possibly the interface to the internal world was being changed as well. After all, the visual system gives the greatest forewarning of impending danger, and appropriate internal reactions such as adrenaline secretion do take place.

The results of this experiment were very rewarding. First, by using simple electrical stimulation of motor cortex, we demonstrated that the motor representation of the trained forearm was also about four times as large as the motor representation, in the other hemisphere, of the untrained forearm. Second, by recording from more than 160 nerve cells, we demonstrated that of all polysensory cells 78 percent responded to somatic stimuli, 54 percent responded to visual stimuli, and 13 percent responded to auditory stimuli. Cells responsive to the orientation of the danger visual stimulus were three times more frequent as other types and many of them also responded to somatic stimulation of the trained forearm.

To my knowledge this is the first time it has been shown that early experience can induce hemispheric asymmetry in animals. I was extremely interested to see if the animals exhibited handedness—the preferred use of one forearm over the other. We ran a large battery of tests that demonstrated that the trained forearm was consistently preferred in reaching or manipulating.

Implications for Infant Stimulation

What these results unequivocally demonstrate is that during certain periods of time after birth large parts of the brain, particularly those at the interface with the external and the internal world, are being configured under the guidance of a variety of stimuli, with the aim of achieving the best possible match for a specific environmental domain. The higher the animal species, the more plasticity and configuring there is. The advantage, naturally, is greater adaptability. The disadvantage is that there is more need for a caregiver who knows how to deliver the best configuration sequence. I use the word *sequence* to imply that timing is as critical as the nature of the information delivered.

This is particularly true of the preterm infant. As many of us at this Round Table have noted, the primary task for the preterm infant is to achieve homeostasis in the face of a large variety of stimuli impinging on systems that are not ready for stimulation. Yet stimuli have to be given to help the infant achieve or maintain homeostasis, to interface with the environment, and to configure his neural/mental potential. In some ways the brain resembles the immunological system—it has to be challenged to achieve proper function. These stimuli are permanently changing, for better or worse, the actual structure of the brain.

The caregiver is unavoidably a brain-shaper who has a very large impact in determining the future learning predispositions of the infant. Seemingly minor experiences, stimuli, and interventions can have very large effects in the future. Most infants turn out all right, in part by sheer luck, in part because of the tremendous investments in time, love, and energy of caregivers. But we need to know more about which stimuli and experiences, given at the critical time, can help infants realize their full potential.

Our experiments with kittens indicate that early transactions with the environment partition neural resources, allocating them to systems involved in those transactions at the expense of other systems. Abilities and disabilities are created simultaneously. (For example, learning Italian as a child does produce a disability in English pronunciation.) Much as we depend on the help of creative architects to achieve a harmonious partitioning of a house while realizing our individual goals, so are children dependent on caregivers in the task of harmoniously partitioning that most precious of all resources, home to the mind, and that is the brain.

DISCUSSION

Anneliese Korner: There has been much talk about whether or not it is good for children to grow up bilingually. In terms of your knowledge, if there's only so much room in the house, what is your guess?

Nico Spinelli: The body uses the resources almost to the fullest. For example, if you put a human being in orbit, calcium will immediately start moving out of the bones—just to show how tight things are in the body/house, so to speak. However, the brain is such an important component that plenty of reserves are kept aside. Coles and a colleague did an experiment in monkeys in which they ablated the motor area corresponding to the thumb. They were very careful not to damage anything else, just the thumb area. The next day the monkey's thumb was paralyzed, but in about two weeks motion came back. When they opened up the head again they found that nearby cortical areas that previously had not caused thumb movement now did. They destroyed those also, and this time the thumb was permanently paralyzed. So there is a reserve sitting there waiting for the brain cells to die off, little blood vessels to clog, and so on. And therefore, people don't realize their full potential. So it's very important to generate a plan right away, rather than leaving it to chance.

To answer your question directly, I think that growing up bilingually wastes real estate in the brain. A better plan, in my opinion, would be for children to learn to pronounce perfectly fifty or so words of, say, German, French, Japanese, and Spanish. Later on, one or more of these languages could be learned more easily and with no accent, because the brain would have been primed for it.

Cynthia Garcia Coll: In your cat experiments, where you gave them a painful stimulus, what would happen if the stimulus were a positive stimulus? Would the brain allocate as much space for something that is positive as for something that is negative? And what would be the implications for positive learning versus negative learning?

Nico Spinelli: If you give cats an aversive stimulus, like an electric shock, it has to be strong enough so that they're not bored by it, but not strong enough that they feel that this is a fighting situation. So our stimulus is aversive but nothing serious. It's true that aversive stimuli are important; you cannot afford to miss the tiger in the jungle, whereas you can afford to walk by the apple tree and get the apple tomorrow. But more important than that is how much information the experience conducts. It doesn't matter how much stimulus you get; it's the information it delivers.

This is why I am sometimes upset at research on the P300 response. It is an indicator, which is good—it gives a feeling that something is going on—but it does not quite capture the situation. If that information is surprising and important, then the organism records it and allocates the resources and changes. But "surprise" and "informative" have to be in the context of what we know. A Stone Age person might not be surprised by a computer terminal. There is a relationship between the knowledge that we have and what is coming in that makes it worth recording.

Peter Gorski: To play with the architectural analogy just one step further, does that conceptual model support those eager parents, or so-called educators, who would, say, prefer their infant child to learn to play the cello before or rather than walking and therefore inculcate it in the experience of the child?

Nico Spinelli: First of all, let me say that I believe in equal worth. We're all human beings.

We know from neurology that different parts of the brain mature at different times, that different types of knowledge impact on different parts of the brain, and that these modifications one produces are irreversible. So if you want to set up an educational program, you have to know when to do it. People who teach singing know about the larynx; they don't start with voice training until the right age. Educators should know about the brain.

Peter Gorski: I wanted to hear you say that.

Craig Ramey: Another education question. The corollary I draw is that if one wanted to provide educational experiences to children who might otherwise not have them, one should examine the experiences that are perhaps most useful for functioning in a particular society or culture or social class. It would seem to me that the argument would lead one to attempt to create a set of experiences that emphasized breadth as well as depth. And the question is, how deep do you have to go? If you have some reason to believe that Chinese is going to be important, how much exposure to Chinese do you need to hold that space, as it were?

Also, do I understand you correctly when I interpret you to mean that enrichment or breadth of experience is an area that you would focus on for children who are at risk for not doing well in whatever set of areas one would deem to be important?

Nico Spinelli: Well, even the computer scientists, the artificial intelligence people, have come up with the idea of domain-specific knowledge. You're absolutely right that depending on the domain, different skills are most important. I was a little too drastic when I said that these changes are permanent. They are very hard to reverse, but certainly you can reclaim some of the territory. What I am really advocating here is something like this: not investing children with the whole ball of wax, if I can say that, but rather creating in them some specific learning predisposition for two or three topics that educators agree are critical. And the point of it all is that you don't need a giant program. You just need a few minutes, maybe once a week. In the case of setting up a learning predisposition for Chinese—one of my favorite examples, actually—I would guess that a few perfectly learned sentences, containing all of the important phonemes, might suffice. At the very least, words learned later would be spoken without accent. Breadth of experience could be more easily achieved by establishing many such "islands of certainty." Our data suggest that this would be better, as a method, than attempting to impart very large amounts of unavoidably ill-defined knowledge.

Jennifer Buchwald: Just a couple of comments with regard to some of the recordings I was talking about with the P300, which by the way is an interesting and objective way of doing a discrimination of two different sounds. You've been stressing the motor aspect, or the production of sound; we were stressing the reception of sound. In most neurobiology, as you were pointing out, the receptive areas not only are represented in the larger area of the cortex, or of the nervous system, but they also mature earlier than the motor counterpart. The individuals that we study can neither discriminate nor produce *r*'s and *l*'s. They say *lice* for *rice* and so forth. In part I think this is because the people who teach English in Japan cannot pronounce English correctly; they make exactly the same mistakes as their students, so the children learning in the schools never hear English pronounced properly.

We think this inability reflects an environmental effect. We're not sure when it starts, but we are predicting that diminished discrimination for some phonemes will start showing up at around ten or twelve years old. Until that point, all nationalities are going to be able to discriminate everything. But one thing we have seen in our data is that there are some individuals who have had no special advantage—they've gone to public schools, they've heard the same mispronunciation of English as everyone else—and yet they can hear these differences. They have a good clear P300 and pronounce the words very well. So people aren't uniform. Some do have unique predilections, a special skill in a particular sensory area such as sound perception.

Nico Spinelli: There is a very well-developed learning theory now concerning what is called super-conditioning. If you have no expectation about something and it happens and you are surprised, it brings you information, and you learn something about it. But if what happens is the opposite of what you were expecting, then your surprise is greater. Then you get super-conditioning. When I show you three vertical bars in one eye, the expectation is that the other eye is going to see three vertical bars too. At least that's what has always happened in my experience. I see the same thing with both eyes. If on the other hand a millisecond or so later you get a completely different experience in the other eye, that is a plasticity-triggering experience, because you are very surprised.

It's a well-known clinical fact that there are some therapists who are much better than some other therapists at getting brain-damaged people to recover. There are teachers who can teach music to a tone-deaf person, and there are some who can't. Yes, people are different, but are *they* different, or are the experiences they get different?

DEVELOPMENT AND PLASTICITY OF THE ASSOCIATION CORTEX

Michael L. Schwartz, Ph.D.,
and Patricia Goldman-Rakic, Ph.D.

Numerous studies over the last three decades (for reviews see Rothblat & Schwartz, 1978; Hubel & Wiesel, 1977) make it clear that sensory areas of the immature brain are susceptible to a variety of forces that play a role in the final determination of their anatomical, functional, and biochemical organization. While our knowledge of the effects of stimulation on sensory and motor regions of the central nervous system has grown, we remain relatively naive about the effects of early stimulation on the association areas of the cerebral cortex. This paper discusses recent research on the developmental and organizational features of the primate prefrontal association cortex. These studies suggest that the development of association areas of the primate cerebral cortex may differ from that of sensory regions.

Research Methods

We chose the monkey prefrontal cortex (PFC) as the focus for these studies for several reasons. First, the cytoarchitecture of prefrontal cortical areas in the monkey brain is more differentiated than that found in any nonprimate species and is in many ways similar to that of the human prefrontal region. Second, damage to the PFC in monkeys produces a pattern of cognitive and behavioral deficits that is in many ways analogous to that found in humans with frontal lobe damage (see Goldman-Rakic et al., 1983, for review). Finally, recent studies (Barbas & Mesulam, 1981; Goldman & Nauta, 1977; Goldman-Rakic & Schwartz, 1982; Jacobson & Trojanowski, 1977a, 1977b; Schwartz & Goldman-Rakic, 1984) have provided detailed information on the connectivity in the adult PFC that may be used as a basis for examining the development and plasticity of this region.

Extensive connections with other cortical areas constitute one of the distinguishing features of the PFC. Studies of cortico-cortical connections in sensory regions of a number of species (Innocenti, 1981; O'Leary et al., 1981; Ivy & Killackey, 1982) suggest that they may be determined in part by characteristics of the early postnatal sensory environment. An understanding of the similarities and differences in development for these connections in different regions of cortex may provide insight into the degree to which they may also be modified by stimulation.

To assess the pattern of cortical connections, we have used a variety of pathway tracing methodologies, which may be generally classed as *anterograde* or *retrograde*. Anterograde tracers are used to visualize the pattern of termination of neurons in an area of interest. When these substances are injected into the brain, they are taken up by the cell bodies and dendrites of neurons in the injected area and transported axonally to the terminal regions of these cells, where they may be examined in histologically processed brain slices. Retrograde tracers are used to visualize the cells that give rise to axons and terminals in a particular area of the brain. These substances are taken up by the terminals of axons in the injected region and transported axonally back to the cells of origin, where they can be examined with histological methods or by viewing brain sections under specific wavelengths of fluorescent illumination (see figure 2). With the use of these methods individually or in combination, it is possible to map the sources and targets of connections of the PFC and to detail their organization within this area.

ANTEROGRADE TRANSPORT

RETROGRADE TRANSPORT

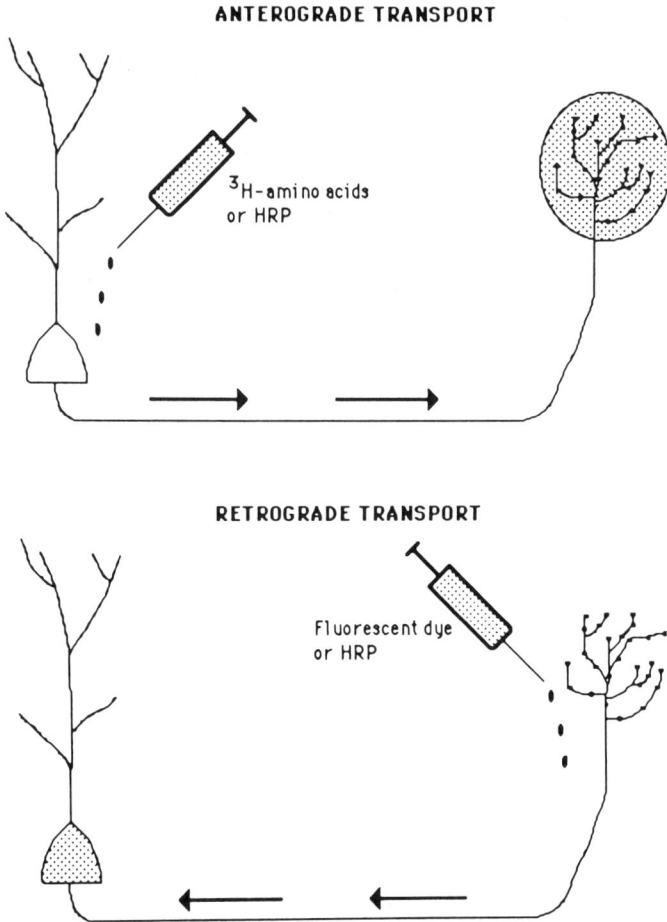

Figure 2. Schematic diagram of anterograde and retrograde tracing paradigms. *Top:* Anterograde transport labels terminal regions of a neuronal population. In this example, tritiated amino acids or HRP are injected into the vicinity of cell bodies whose region of termination is of interest. The tracer is taken up by the soma and dendrites of these cells and transported through the axon to the terminal region of the cells (stippled area), where it is visualized through autoradiographic methods (with ^{3}H-amino acids) or histochemical methods (with HRP). *Bottom:* Retrograde transport identifies the neuronal origin of axons and terminals within an area of interest. Here tracers are injected in the area of interest and transported intra-axonally to the cell bodies (stippled) that have terminals in the injected area. Cells labeled by the tracer are then visualized histochemically (with HRP) or in a microscope equipped with a fluorescent illuminator (with fluorescent dyes).

Organization of Cortico-Cortical Connections in the Adult Monkey

Studies of the organization of prefrontal connectivity in the adult monkey indicate:

1. Cortico-cortical neurons and their terminal territories are organized in a modular or columnar pattern. For example, if we inject anterograde tracers into the posterior parietal cortex of one hemisphere and examine the pattern of termination in the PFC of the same hemisphere, the regions of termination appear as vertically oriented columns about a half millimeter in width, alternating with unlabeled regions of approximately the same size (Goldman-Rakic & Schwartz, 1982; Schwartz & Goldman-Rakic, 1984). Injection into areas of the opposite hemisphere that project to the PFC via the corpus callosum also reveals a columnar pattern of termination with similar dimensions (Goldman & Nauta, 1977). If we examine the organization of neurons which give rise to these columns of terminals by injecting retrograde tracers into the PFC, we seldom see sharply demarcated columns of cells (Schwartz & Goldman-Rakic, 1984), but careful quantitative analysis also reveals a modular organization in the density distribution of these neurons.

2. The columns of divergent afferent and efferent domains occupy unique and interdigitated territories within the PFC (Goldman-Rakic & Schwartz, 1982; Schwartz & Goldman-Rakic, 1984). To demonstrate this pattern of organization, we injected anterograde tracers into two different sources of cortical input to the principal sulcus (PS) of the PFC (see figure 3a). This paradigm revealed that ipsilateral and contralateral inputs terminate in separate and alternating columnar territories (figure 3b).

3. The adult pattern of connectivity is characterized by a radial organization in which terminals arising from other cortical areas (afferent connections) and the projection cells of the PFC (efferent connections) are differentially distributed among the six layers of the cortex.

Development of Cortico-Cortical Connectivity

Our studies into the development of prefrontal cortico-cortical connections were designed to provide basic information on the

3a.

3b.

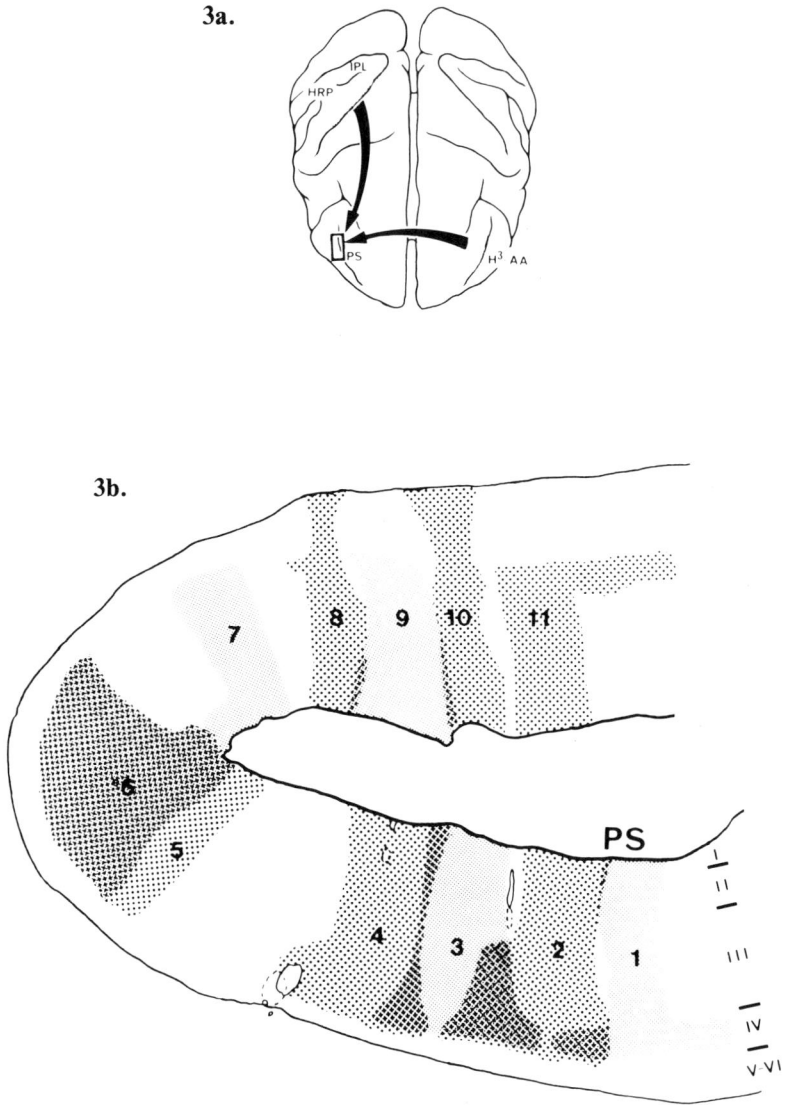

Figure 3. Composite diagram of two adjacent sections from the principal sulcus (PS) in the prefrontal cortex. *a.* HRP was injected into the inferior parietal lobule (IPL) of the same hemisphere, and ^{3}H-amino acids were injected into the PFC of the opposite hemisphere. The outlined box indicates the area of cortex examined. *b.* Autoradiographically labeled callosal fiber columns (2, 4, 5, 8, 10, and 11) are indicated by the coarse stipple; associational fiber columns (1, 3, 6, 7, and 9) originating from the parietal cortex, labeled by anterograde transport of HRP, are shown as fine stipple.

timetables for the establishment of afferent and efferent connections in the PFC and to assess the rules and mechanisms that guide this development. Among the issues we wanted to address were these:

1. Is the modular pattern of cortico-cortical neuron and terminal domains sculpted from an initially diffuse and uniform distribution? For example, studies in sensory cortices of rats and cats indicate that neurons projecting through the corpus callosum in immature animals are distributed uniformly throughout these areas. In contrast, these cells have a restricted or uneven distribution in the same areas in mature animals. Only gradually during postnatal development does the columnar or modular distribution emerge. In the case of the visual cortex, the eventual pattern of connectivity in the mature animal appears to be due at least in part to early visual stimulation (Innocenti, Frost, & Illes, 1985).

2. Do neurons of the PFC have a more widespread pattern of connectivity in the immature animal than in the adult? If so, is environmental stimulation important in shaping the eventual pattern? Studies of sensory cortex in cats and rats have identified transient cortico-cortical connections in the neonate that are not found in the mature brain (Innocenti & Clarke, 1984).

To assess the pattern of development in the PFC, we injected fetal and postnatal monkeys with anterograde and retrograde tracers to determine the pattern of connectivity at various points in development. Fetal monkeys of known gestational age were briefly exteriorized by an incision in the uterus, injected, and returned to the uterus for two to ten days to allow transport of the tracers in the pathways under investigation.

The earliest age examined was embryonic day 82 (E82) of the 165-day gestational period. At this stage only an occasional neuron within the PFC is labeled by injection of retrograde tracers into its prospective targets. Between E100 and E124 cortico-cortical neurons both within the PFC and in areas projecting to the PFC begin to emerge in large numbers. During this period all cortical areas that project to the PFC in mature monkeys contained labeled neurons, and we found no labeled neurons in areas that do not project to the PFC in adults. Assessment of the laminar and columnar distribution of cortico- cortical neurons in these same monkeys revealed that these organizational features also appear in a mature form a full month prior to birth.

Studies of the terminal distribution of cortical inputs to the PFC were also examined by placing injections of anterograde tracers into the PFC of the opposite hemisphere (Goldman-Rakic, 1981). The results of these experiments revealed that the columnar organization of these connections is apparent from the time of ingrowth of these axons into the cortex, at least one month prior to birth. These studies of developing afferents and efferents suggest that there is a relatively high degree of specificity involved in the formation of cortico-cortical connections of the primate prefrontal cortex.

Summary

The results of our studies of cortico-cortical connectivity in developing monkey association cortex contrast with those obtained in comparable studies of sensory regions in other species. In association areas these connections emerge very early in development, and many of the details of their organization are well specified from their earliest appearance. The presence of an adult-like pattern of organization a full month before birth suggests that these events are probably determined in large part by forces independent of general environmental stimulation. One interpretation of our results could be that diverse areas of the cerebral cortex may differ in the extent to which they respond to environmental influences. However, we should not completely rule out the possibility that since many of the features of connectional organization that are responsive to the environment in the sensory areas (for example, the distribution of cortico-cortical neurons) develop during the prenatal period in the PFC they may simply be buffered from the effects of environmental stimuli. In addition, other aspects of the circuitry of the prefrontal cortex clearly continue to develop well into the postnatal period and may be subject to modification by experience. Among these are the organization and density of synaptic contacts (Bourgeois et al., 1985) and the elaboration of dendritic surfaces (Cupp & Uemura, 1980). Although relatively little is known concerning the response of these parameters to stimulation in the PFC, studies from sensory areas suggest that these may be good candidates for modification by external interventions.

DISCUSSION

Nico Spinelli: The word *association* is broad. Some people call association cortices *polysensory cortices,* and in the monkey you do have cortical areas that are part of an intrinsic system. They have no connection with the outside world, so to speak, whereas the extrinsic system does. So your argument, as I understand it, is that you see no plasticity, because the intrinsic system does not have to adapt to the outside world, whereas the extrinsic system does, and therefore plasticity is useful there.

Michael Schwartz: I am saying that our data on the timing and developmental emergence of cortico-cortical connections in the primate PFC indicate that early on these connections do not appear to have the same type of exuberance of targets and neuronal distribution that they exhibit in sensory areas. Further, a full month prior to birth their radial and tangential distribution is similar to that found in adult monkeys. Since it is these organizational features that mature during the postnatal period and appear to be modified by environmental conditions of stimulation in the sensory areas of the cerebral cortex, our data would suggest that these connections in the association areas are probably insulated from environmental modification. This is not to say that all aspects of the circuitry of the prefrontal cortex are fixed. As I have indicated, some features of the connectivity of the PFC are undoubtedly modified during the postnatal period. Further, you might conceive that the modifications of sensory areas may confer a functional plasticity on the association areas just by the altered patterns of input they offer for processing to these areas. What I would like to emphasize is that differences in the timing and patterns of development in sensory and association areas may result in a differential susceptibility to modification of the various structural features of these areas.

Nico Spinelli: I've got to accept the evidence, the connections were less variable, but could it be that they were not being challenged in the proper way?

Michael Schwartz: One way to test this would be to lesion one of the adjacent columnar systems early in the development and look for an expansion of the columns of the remaining input. This type of experiment is currently in progress, and only very preliminary results are available from one monkey, but this monkey's system has been challenged in a way very similar to that used in the analysis of sensory system development, and unlike what one might expect, those columns retain their rather mature-looking form.

Berry Brazelton: We see that a baby in a certain state will respond in a certain way, and in another state the same stimulus will cause a disorganized response. Then you see a baby that's impaired or at high risk because of prematurity, immaturity, or stress, and the same stress that will organize a full-term or a well-organized baby will disorganize this baby. I wonder about what we call appropriate stimulation versus inappropriate stimulation, and what that does to this association cortex and its organization.

Michael Schwartz: We have a problem when we look in the association cortex. We don't have the intuitive knowledge of what the proper stimuli or events are for stimulating the neurons within the prefrontal cortex. It's very difficult for us to do the same types of experiments that have been done in sensory areas, where you intuitively have some idea of what a receptive field is like, and what it might be to modify it.

Robert Isaacson: It is possible that the "tuning" of neural systems may involve a different kind of interaction than anybody has talked about yet, in particular the role of some of the peripheral hormones, even in minute quantities, as they exert important influences on the brain. A very small amount of a peripheral hormone in a brain-damaged animal can produce a quite different effect from that found in a normal animal. We are just beginning to recognize the prodigious influences of neuropeptides and neurohormones.

Edward Tronick: As a developmental psychologist, I see the stimulation, the input, as doing a lot of the structuring of the system. Is there also damage coming from inappropriate stimulation? If we're talking about fine-tuning neural systems, no one here has spoken of fine-tuning the system in a negative way, disrupting the system.

Jennifer Buchwald: We don't talk about the development of a complete system any more, because we know that the different sensory systems develop at different rates, and different levels of the brain are integrating information in different ways at different times. Certainly in an adult nervous system, if you overstimulate—for instance, if you give too much auditory stimulation—you get temporary threshold shifts that are very well documented. I don't think that this has been looked at so much in very immature nervous systems, but we do know that generally the immature system is more fragile to stimulation. The recovery cycles are somewhat longer, so that the chances of overstimulating an auditory pathway, for instance, might be greater in that period of immaturity. But at least some of the projection pathways within the auditory system mature very rapidly. In other subcomponents, the system doesn't mature as rapidly. So even within just one system, there are many different parallel pathways at different levels, maturing at different rates.

Berry Brazelton: Could "affect-flooded" be the same as "surprise"? In other words, if you have a positive learning model from having the baby in the proper state and giving him an affect-flooded stimulus, would you be likely to get your response more easily than you would if it were a negative or unimportant stimulus?

Jennifer Buchwald: We haven't explored that, but it would be interesting to try to introduce that into the experimental design. We only know that if the modality is being attended to, if there is something rewarding about attending to the modality, the response occurs.

Peter Vietze: One of the questions that both Ed and Berry asked is whether you can do harm. What dimension of harm are you talking about? As there are multiple levels internally in the brain that could count for various reactions or structures, there are also various dimensions on which you could consider harm: affective harm, cognitive harm, structural harm.

Edward Tronick: It's important to keep these distinctions in mind. I don't mean to underestimate them. But what I meant in a more general sense is that to some extent we are hearing something not unlike a model of some of the processes of normal development. Certainly one of the concerns that brings us all together is the question whether in inappropriate contexts, if there are inappropriate contexts around this process of development, you can take that process of development and derail it because of inappropriate kinds of inputs. Think about the sensory system. Could you recruit sensory fields early on to, say, visual stimuli in the environment by exposing an organism, during that normal period of time when the set-up process is going on, to stimuli that are aberrant in its normal ecology? After all, vertical and horizontal bars are not the typical things that your organisms would encounter. To use Nico's metaphor, would you end up devoting too much of the house to that kind of function and therefore preclude certain other normal functions?

Peter Gorski: I want us to think beyond what may be good or bad to the concepts of adaptive or maladaptive within the environment or the cultural context in which the organism finds itself having to survive and thrive. And this is particularly pertinent to the Round Table as we move toward the clinical research side. For example, do premature infants in the intensive care nursery environment adapt autonomically or in state organization in order to cope with and even survive that extrauterine environment, which they then lose when they go home and are placed into a very different contextual field? At home they will be raised according to wholly different guidelines, and wholly different structure and function in the various neurological systems responsible for adaptation will be encouraged. Given the power of your work suggesting that early influences may set the stage for function later on, or a capacity to learn later on, are we training any of these neurological functions or behavioral functions in ways that will be adaptive only for the short run but in some instances maladaptive over time?

Michael Schwartz: As you know, one thing we've learned from the studies of the sensory systems and their modifiability is that there is a critical period when you can make these modifications. I think we need to address this issue for each type of stimulation that we intend to impose on the premature infant. Take temperature regulation. If we ask this infant to maintain its own temperature, are we asking the system to train itself to do something before it's ready to do that? For example, is there maybe not a biological clock that ticks off at birth to allow the infant to regulate its temperature properly? If so, challenging the system to perform this task before this point would be fruitless and endanger the survival of the infant. One has to be a little cautious about challenging the system of these premature infants to do something that the genetic machinery isn't ready for it to do yet.

PART II

STIMULATION: PSYCHOLOGICAL AND BEHAVIORAL PERSPECTIVES

HANDLING PRETERM INFANTS IN HOSPITALS: STIMULATING CONTROVERSY ABOUT TIMING STIMULATION

Peter A. Gorski, M.D.,
Lee Huntington, Ph.D.,
and David J. Lewkowicz, Ph.D.

Preterm infants are unusual patients. They present hospital professionals with the unique situation of demanding intensive medical care for an essentially healthy organism. Indeed, most of these neonates are born free of organic pathology, yet they have significant organ system immaturities. Inside a well-functioning uterine environment, these infants would likely continue to thrive toward normal outcome at term. Delivered to the extrauterine world of a hospital intensive care nursery (ICN), they are helpless to sustain their own basic life support systems. The cumulative stress of surviving in this environment can take a heavy toll in the form of acquired disease or disabilities. Most medical and developmental risks resulting from premature birth stem from the immature organism's limited ability to adapt to the caregiving environment outside the womb.

We do not necessarily fault medicine's inability to replicate the intrauterine environment. That would probably not even be the best goal. Once born, preterm infants must suddenly activate operations responsible for respiration, thermoregulation, digestion, and motility against gravity, to name the most basic. The caregiving environment, then, must provide the kind and level of support needed to protect the boundaries or vulnerabilities of the organism while simultaneously stimulating further growth and development. The first goal for all concerned should perhaps be a comprehensive understanding of the ontogeny of structure and function of crucial organ systems in preterm infants born at various gestational maturities. Therapeutic interventions performed in the best interest of these atypical infants could then rise from empirically tested conceptual frameworks concerning the integrative capacities of this unique population born too underdeveloped to sustain their original health.

Our own research is primarily concerned with the effects of the caregiving environment upon brain growth and central nervous system (CNS) organization in hospitalized preterm infants. The CNS controls the function of other vital organ systems. Reciprocally, perfusion and resultant oxygenation of brain tissue is affected by changes in systemic circulation. Clinical neonatal medical practice does not routinely monitor fluctuations in cerebral perfusion or, in many cases, even peripheral oxygenation.

To demonstrate the potential value of monitoring caregiving effects on CNS functioning in preterm infants, we study the relationship between trends in physiological distress signs and a variety of caregiving interventions. In a previous Round Table presentation (Gorski et al., 1984), we reported the earliest findings from our San Francisco study of preterm infant and caregiver behavior. The current report summarizes the initial analyses completed using the entire study sample collected during 1983 and 1984. We will discuss physiological trends in preterm infant heart rate and oxygenation as related to timing and content of caregiver stimulation.

Specifically, we examined the amounts and types of touch (medical and social) in a group of hospitalized preterm infants and how these forms of touch related to a particular physiological crisis—bradycardia (low heart rate)—in these infants. In addition, we explored the relationship of heart rate and oxygenation status to the occurrence of bradycardic episodes. Finally, we examined the relationship of these physiologic indices to bradycardia in the presence and absence of caregiver touch. It is important to note that these results represent suggestive evidence limited by the small sample available for analysis from this pilot study.

The Research Method

Eighteen preterm infants hospitalized in the Intensive Care Nursery at Mount Zion Hospital and Medical Center in San Francisco were observed twice weekly for three weeks or until their hospital discharge. The neonates studied were born between 28 and 34 weeks' gestational age (mean=31 weeks), and observations began in their second week of life. They were born appropriate weight for gestational age, had no congenital anomalies or infections, and were convalescent following initial acute illness. They were off ventilator, breathing room air, and tolerating tube or nipple feedings.

Observations lasted an average of 208 minutes, between morning and early afternoon. They were naturalistically recorded without altering nursery routine. Observers were trained in the use of an original premature infant behavioral observation scale (High & Gorski, 1985). Data were collected at the infant's bedside in the ICN with a small, cart-mounted microcomputer system (for details about this system, see Gorski et al., 1983), which automatically monitored and entered physiologic data and timing and allowed the observer to enter coded data on a keyboard. Every thirty seconds the computer recorded and displayed transcutaneous pO_2 and heart rate, while the observer entered data on such behavioral observations as sleep/wake state, skin color, activity level, medical procedures, social care, feeding, grooming, persons in attendance, ambient environmental stimuli, and infant responses and expressions.

At the time of the study, cardiac deceleration below 100 beats per minute (BPM) was considered clinically significant. Monitor alarms were set to sound at heart rates less than 100 BPM, and caregivers routinely noted and responded to such episodes. For our purposes we therefore defined bradycardia as a recorded heart rate under 100 BPM.

The observation periods were divided into five-minute periods and classified either as baseline periods—all five-minute periods except those immediately preceding bradycardic episodes—and pre-bradycardic periods—those five-minute periods preceding the occurrence of a bradycardic episode. Each period was further classified on the basis of whether or not touch occurred during that time.

Results

Of the eighteen infants observed, ten had episodes of bradycardia and eight did not. The ten who had bradycardic episodes collectively had forty episodes. Of these, thirteen (32 percent) were associated with at least one episode of touch in the preceding five minutes, and 27 (68 percent) had no touch in the preceding five minutes. Eight of the ten infants had at least one pre-bradycardic period that contained touch. Seven had at least one pre-bradycardic period with no touch. Five had both touch and no-touch pre-bradycardic periods.

Most instances of bradycardia in this sample thus did not appear to be associated with touch. Moreover, there was no statistically significant difference in the occurrence of touch in pre-bradycardic periods and in baseline periods for the ten bradycardic infants, indicating that handling does not automatically lead to cardiac instability.

Six of the thirteen episodes associated with touch followed tracheal suctioning, a particularly stressful procedure. In the remaining episodes, the ratio of medical to social touch was the same as the baseline rate. This finding suggests that efforts at "developmental stimulation" or social interaction, if poorly timed, could stress a vulnerable infant as much as medical procedures.

Neither absolute heart rate values nor trends in heart rate prior to bradycardia appeared to predict the occurrence of bradycardia, either overall or in relation to touch. This finding is particularly provocative considering that heart rate monitoring is a nearly universal, and often singular, standard of clinical practice in ICNs.

In contrast, however, transcutaneous oxygen monitoring added significant information. While there were no differences between the baseline $TcPO_2$ values of those infants who had bradycardic episodes and those who did not, there was a marginal change in $TcPO_2$ over five minutes prior to bradycardia.

When the presence or absence of touch was added to the examination of $TcPO_2$ levels, an interesting pattern of results emerged. First, the pre-bradycardic periods without touch had significantly higher than baseline $TcPO_2$ values at the beginning, which then decreased toward the end of the period preceding bradycardia. This result may reveal the operation of a compensatory mechanism. It may be, for example, that in response to central hypoventilation or hypoperfusion, the infant attempts to hyperventilate or increase heart rate but is unable to sustain the effort, with resultant fatigue or sudden autonomic collapse.

$TcPO_2$ was marginally lower throughout those pre-bradycardic periods that included touch than in the baseline periods. While this result suggests that touch may lower $TcPO_2$ and thereby precipitate a bradycardic episode, $TcPO_2$ was the same for the touch and no-touch baselines. This finding argues that touch by itself does not necessarily lower $TcPO_2$ but may contribute to bradycardia when the infant is already physiologically compromised with low $TcPO_2$. The touch may also represent a caregiver's response to signs of distress in an infant.

While bradycardia and hypoxemia occur relatively infrequently in hospitalized infants, such crises must be regarded seriously by developmentalists as well as by cardiopulmonary specialists. Events such as apnea, bradycardia, and hypoxemia can trigger or involve changes in cerebral autoregulation of blood flow, intracranial pressure, cerebral oxygen, and carbon dioxide tension, putting these infants at risk for postnatal intraventricular hemorrhage or infarction. Our aim is to determine ways in which our caregiving observations and interventions could protect preterm infants from such occurrences. We believe our work already points out the need to reconsider current methods of clinical physiological monitoring to highlight not only absolute values but potentially critical trends that might precede significant distress. As for developmental implications, we trust our findings support an orientation toward and respect for maturational stages and times of vulnerability as well as receptivity to sensory input in preterm infants. It is our hope that such considerations will serve as conceptual anchors and empirical tests for developmental stimulation programs in the future.

DISCUSSION

Frances Horowitz: Peter, do you think that there are individual differences, that for some infants touch is a more destabilizing stimulus than for other infants? If you observe the same infant over a period of time, do you notice that there are some modalities of stimulation that are more beneficial and some that are more disruptive? Would that be a useful strategy to pursue?

Peter Gorski: Well, I would hate to say yes, even if that were true, because then people would apply blanket concepts of intervention: something will always benefit this infant and something else will never benefit this infant. I think maturational stages influence whether or not a particular effort is stabilizing or destabilizing. Yes, there are individual differences among babies. I'm becoming more and more convinced, however, that conditions and not the baby's individual traits are predictive of whether or not an intervention will be stabilizing or destabilizing.

Barry Lester: If it's true that medical and caregiving interventions affect $TcPO_2$ or heart rate, how meaningful are those kinds of short-term changes? Are you seriously concerned that you are going to create an intraventricular hemorrhage or other problems?

Peter Gorski: Yes, I am seriously concerned, as are others, that we are unintentionally but daily fracturing little blood vessels in the brains of babies. We know now from ultrasound studies—Nelson in Chicago in particular has been doing this work with Birnholz—that unless you measure ultrasound serially every week, you will find that holes in the brain created by bleed or infarction can completely disappear, resorb. The brain matter will look entirely normal two weeks later, and you would never notice it, but later on the child may turn out to have spastic motor problems. Yes, there is concern that these small perturbations are in fact having long-lasting effects but may not even be evidenced for a while, or may come and go. It just makes eminent sense that if hypoxemia in the peripheral circulation is associated with compensatory changes, systemic blood pressure goes up. With increased systemic blood pressure, intracranial pressure goes up. There's an alteration of the autoregulatory capacity within the cerebral vasculature, so cerebral blood flow rates go up, and pulse pressure changes increase within the brain. Given the fragile nature of these capillaries, that's about the best explanation that any of us has right now for the occurrence of postnatal intraventricular hemorrhage.

Peter Vietze: Peter, you said that there probably are individual differences in how these babies would react to different kinds of stimulation, but you wouldn't want it to be known that something works with one and something else doesn't work. I don't understand why not. It would seem to me that you would want to design an optimal program, so you know that for Baby A these things work and will do some good and these things don't work and also may do harm.

Peter Gorski: Well, first of all, it's because I can't say as a fact that such individual differences exist. And secondly, I believe that they will turn out to be less important considerations than the conditions—the physiological and environmental conditions—about the baby at the time any intervention is considered. Whether the intervention is routine or developmental or medical, I believe these conditions might be better predictors of the effect of the intervention as stabilizing or destabilizing.

Arthur Parmelee: Babies change day by day, as a function of biological maturation and environmental inputs. A measure of a baby's neurological organization would give you a clue as to what environmental inputs the baby could tolerate. Stimulation would then depend on what's going on within and around the baby and how physiologically stable the baby can be in these circumstances. Stimuli the baby might tolerate one day very successfully could be overwhelming the next day. We aren't yet able to anticipate these variations in responsiveness.

Peter Vietze: So you're saying that because of daily changes in conditions you could never design a plan for a baby?

Arthur Parmelee: Plans are necessary to set guidelines based on information we are now discussing, but there should be some adaptations of the plan for each baby daily. We should avoid ritual interventions based on a rigid plan.

Peter Gorski: I'm particularly interested in studying intervention opportunities that are based on observation of the baby's condition and the course of events around the baby that day, rather than putting out a handbook that says all babies who are 32 weeks' conceptual age benefit from this kind of stimulation at ten o'clock in the morning.

Frances Horowitz: Are you implying that at 32 weeks of age there are differences between babies that would suggest that one would tailor the intervention? that for some babies touch is a more disorganizing stimulus than for other babies, and that with some babies you back off and reduce the amount of certain kinds of stimulation, while other babies can handle more? The question is whether these are stable individual differences. I don't know that we know the answer to that, but if they were, then you could put into the equation the conditions plus the individual differences and get a better outcome.

Peter Gorski: Indeed. Let me just add one more word. Babies of 32 weeks' gestational age, for instance, are at a variety of maturational points. Thirty-two weeks does not imply a certain maturation level for all babies.

Nico Spinelli: Are there guidelines on how much a baby is touched, or with what kind of touches, or is it simply done as needed by the nursing staff?

Peter Gorski: There are no guidelines. Each staff develops its own notions, and some have stated policies while others don't. I think that we're all coming to agree that protection for the smallest and most fragile babies may be the best part of developmental intervention or stimulation.

Barry Nurcombe: Bradycardia, I gather, means "slowing" rather than "slow." Is there evidence that bradycardia is an index of a pathological condition?

Peter Gorski: We polled all the eminent neonatologists at the Cardiovascular Research Institute in San Francisco. No two of them could agree on what represented absolute levels of pathology or life threat with respect to heart rate or oxygenation status. What they all agreed, however, was that at this time they were unwilling to let a heart rate of 100 BPM go unnoticed and unresponded to.

Barry Nurcombe: But is there any evidence that it's a dangerous state to be in?

Peter Gorski: No, that's why I feel that our work and other work like it has an opportunity to help the cardiopulmonary effort of neonatal medicine.

Barry Nurcombe: In these bradycardic babies, once oxygen got above a certain level, that might be a signal that things were going awry. Is that right?

Peter Gorski: Yes, that's of great interest. But again, the current electronic monitoring systems of signaling an absolute point of heart rate or oxygen or respiration are very profound indicators of distress and very nonspecific.

Edward Tronick: Are these stressors what they seem to be? Below 100 BPM is considered a bradycardic episode, and apnea episodes are considered pathological. But are they damaging? I think there's now some feeling that there may be some normal apnea.

Peter Gorski: And that apnea may not be predictive of sudden infant death syndrome (SIDS). Some apnea may conceivably protect the organism from SIDS.

Edward Tronick: Which brings up a much larger point, something that Bob talked about yesterday. I think we assume that optimal care is stressless. But there are many models that require stress, what Nico called *challenges,* in order for development to occur. We may want to reframe this in other terms.

Peter Gorski: I think our interventions over time will need to be conceived in such a manner that we think about protecting the boundaries of the developing nervous system at the same time that we stimulate the capacities within that system.

STATE ORGANIZATION IN PRETERM INFANTS: MICROANALYSIS OF 24-HOUR POLYGRAPHIC RECORDINGS

**James A. Garbanati, Ph.D.,
and Arthur H. Parmelee, M.D.**

It is generally recognized that neonatal infants behave and respond to stimulation differently in different states of sleep and wakefulness (Prechtl & Beintema, 1964; Wolff, 1966; Emde & Koenig, 1969; Korner, 1969; Brazelton, 1973; Prechtl, 1974). It is therefore important to define states and state changes in neonatal infants during any evaluation of spontaneous behaviors or interactions with environmental stimuli. With preterm infants, the problem of defining states is particularly difficult because of the immaturity of their nervous systems. Yet an understanding of the level of their state organization at each age as they mature is crucial to our understanding of their behavioral development and their potential for environmental interaction.

Although there have been a number of studies of state organization in preterm neonates, they have been based on recordings of limited duration, and the analyses of the polygraphic data have been of limited complexity. The study of the development of state organization is currently gaining renewed attention because of new technology that permits the long-term recording of state parameters and facilitates managing the massive amount of data obtained. In this paper, two examples from an ongoing study involving long-term polygraphical recordings of preterm infants are used to illustrate the complexity of state organization and the potential usefulness of some forms of microanalytic studies.

The Meaning of State

The term *state* has many meanings, and this has created confusion among those studying neonatal infant behavior. Prechtl and Beintema (1964) proposed using the term *state* to describe constellations of certain functional patterns and physiological variables that may be relatively stable and that seem to repeat themselves. This definition, which makes clear that one parameter is not sufficient to define a state, has been particularly useful to us. In studies of infants with immature systems and limited state organization, it is imperative to use multiple parameters in order to be able to identify the organizing or disorganizing effects of biological and environmental events.

In earlier concepts, states of sleep and wakefulness were seen as being on a continuum of arousal, from deep sleep to light sleep and on up to various levels of wakefulness. The current concept is that states are discontinuous, separately organized neurological entities within which there can be different levels of arousal, especially during waking.

The Parameters of State

At present the decision regarding which variables and how many to use varies among investigators and is the source of much of the variation in reported findings. For our microanalytic studies of the development of state organization, we consider variability of heart rate and respiration and movements of the eyes and body to be particularly important state parameters for preterm infants.

Table 1 summarizes our criteria for the various states.

Table 1   Sleep/Wake State Criteria

State Category	Respiratory Variability	Heart Rate Variability	Eye Movement	Body Movement	Crying	Eyes Open
ACTIVE SLEEP	high	high	+	Frequent trunk and/or limb movements	+, – (not sustained)	+, – (< 2 minutes consecutively)
QUIET SLEEP	low	low	–	Brief limb twitches, little or no trunk and limb movement	–	
TRANSITION	One Discrepant Variable Occurs					
WAKE STATE	0	0	0	Continuous movement (>1 minute consecutively)	+ (sustained)	+ (>1 minute consecutively)

State in Preterm Neonates

Studies of the ontogeny of state organization in preterm infants have increased our general understanding of sleep and wakefulness in infants. The youngest viable infants appear to have no consistently identifiable states of sleep or wakefulness. Periods of quiescence and activity occur first in body and eye movements and later in heart rate and respiratory rate variability. Gradually the quiescent and active phases of each parameter begin occurring together in predictable sequences for significant periods of time and can be identified as specific states. In general, such well-defined organization of states is found to take place sometime between 34 and 38 weeks' conceptional age (Parmelee & Stern, 1972).

In the youngest preterm infants, 24 to 27 weeks' conceptional age, movements are frequent, including diffuse jerks, localized twitches, and clonic perioral facial movements (Dreyfus-Brisac, 1968). These seem to have limited influence on heart rate or respiratory variability. Heart rate tends to be semiregular, and respirations mostly irregular (Watanabe, Iwase, & Hara, 1973). Eye movements are present but scattered and seldom occur in bursts. Crying is infrequent and unsustained (Dreyfus-Brisac, 1968). After 30 weeks' conceptional age, there is a gradual decline in gross body movements and, to a lesser extent, in localized movements until 35 to 38 weeks' conceptional age (Dreyfus-Brisac, 1970; Prechtl et al., 1979; Fukumoto et al., 1981; Peirano et al., 1986). Then there is a significant decrease in all movements regardless of state. How much of the decrease in movement at this conceptional age is a function of the development of quiet sleep rather than a function of a more general suppression of body movements independent of state remains a question. In all studies there seem to be major changes in the amount of movement in the period that would be, for the fetus, the last month of pregnancy, when there is known to be a drop in fetal movement.

The respirations of preterm infants become increasingly regular with longer and more frequent periods of regular respiration from 32 to 40 weeks' conceptional age. These regular respirations occur more frequently in association with the absence of body movement and eye movements, particularly after 36 weeks (Parmelee & Stern, 1972; Prechtl et al., 1979). Heart rate shows limited variation in the youngest preterms regardless of changes in other parameters, but with maturation there is an increase in variability of heart rate in association with movements and respirations. Heart rate also becomes progressively more closely associated with all the parameters of state (Watanabe, Iwase, & Hara, 1973).

Preterm infants' movement reponses to auditory stimulation do not show any state differences before 34 or 35 weeks' conceptional age, but there is a marked drop in the number of movement responses in quiet sleep from that age to term, while the responses in active sleep remain the same at all ages (Monod & Garma, 1971). This supports the concept of the stimulus-modulating effect of quiet sleep on movement responses. Auditory cortical evoked potentials in term infants have larger amplitudes in the late components in quiet sleep than in active sleep, while in preterm infants before 36 weeks the reverse is often true, suggesting an underdevelopment of state organization in the younger preterm infants (Akiyama et al., 1969). Organized states therefore provide stability against disruption of physiological homeostasis by environmental stimuli in the more mature preterm infants, while very immature preterm infants with no or minimal state organization are vulnerable to environmental stimulation.

Examples of Prolonged Recording of State

In our study we record EKG, respirations, body and eye movements, and caregiving interventions for 24 to 48 hours at weekly intervals. The EKG and respirations are recorded from the electrodes routinely being used to monitor the infant, and body movements from a pressure-sensitive mattress. These data are digitized immediately in a crib-side computer and stored in digital form on a disk. Two video cameras continuously record the infant's behaviors and caregiving procedures, using a time-lapse video recorder, and these data are later scored for eye and body movements and type of caregiving.

We are primarily interested in studying the ontogeny of state organization in each infant. Our expectation is that some of the very young healthy preterm infants will have short periods during the day or night when they have well-organized states, but these states will not be sustained for long periods and will be vulnerable to environmental and biological stresses. Then with maturation there will be a steady increase in the time that organized states are sustained. These sustained organized states will make the infant less vulnerable to stress. On the other hand, preterm infants who have suffered significant perinatal problems are expected to take longer to develop organized states. Increased state organization will then be viewed as a sign of recovery from illness and of nervous system maturation, while continued lack of state organization or the dissolution of previous state organization will be viewed as an indication of continued or developing illness.

Figures 4 and 5 show 24-hour profile plots of two preterm infants, neither of whom ever had significant illness in the neonatal intensive care unit (NICU). The infant represented by figure 4 had a gestational age of 31 weeks and a birthweight of 1,400 grams. He was recorded at 33 and 34 weeks' conceptional age. The infant in figure 5 had a gestational age of 29 weeks and a birthweight of 1,430 grams. He was recorded at 31 and 32 weeks' conceptional age. The first infant continued throughout his nursery stay without any difficulties. The second infant developed some symptoms shortly after the first recording that caused concern about developing necrotizing enterocolitis (NEC), and he was treated for this and possible sepsis for the following week. No definite symptoms of NEC or sepsis materialized, and he was well by the time of the second recording a week later.

The state parameters displayed in figures 4 and 5 are heart rate, heart rate variability (HRV), respiratory rate, respiratory rate variability (RRV), body movements, and eye movements. The filled-in portions of the curves of HRV and RRV represent those segments of these signals that were considered low variability and used to classify quiet sleep. Each plot point is an integration of five minutes of recording. The recording extended from 9:00 a.m. one day to 9:00 a.m. the next day. (Blank spaces indicate periods during which the data were either not available or not scorable.)

The infant whose profile is illustrated in figure 4 was able at 33 weeks' conceptional age to organize multiple short epochs of quiet sleep, representing 12 percent of the scorable record, with active sleep 33 percent, awake 7 percent, and indeterminate state 47 percent. (We have used the term *indeterminate state* rather than *transitional state*, because it is defined by default—that is, it does not reach the criteria for quiet or active sleep or the waking state—even though it occurs most commonly during transition.) A week later, at 34 weeks' conceptional age, there seems to be a more uniform distribution of quiet and active sleep throughout the day. The distributions were quiet sleep 14 percent, active sleep 38 percent, awake 5 percent, and indeterminate state 43 percent. These were not major changes in state organization, though there was somewhat more quiet sleep and active sleep and less indeterminate state.

The younger infant, whose profile is illustrated in figure 5, had at 31 weeks' conceptional age 9 percent quiet sleep, 31 percent active sleep, 15 percent awake, and 45 percent indeterminate state. The main

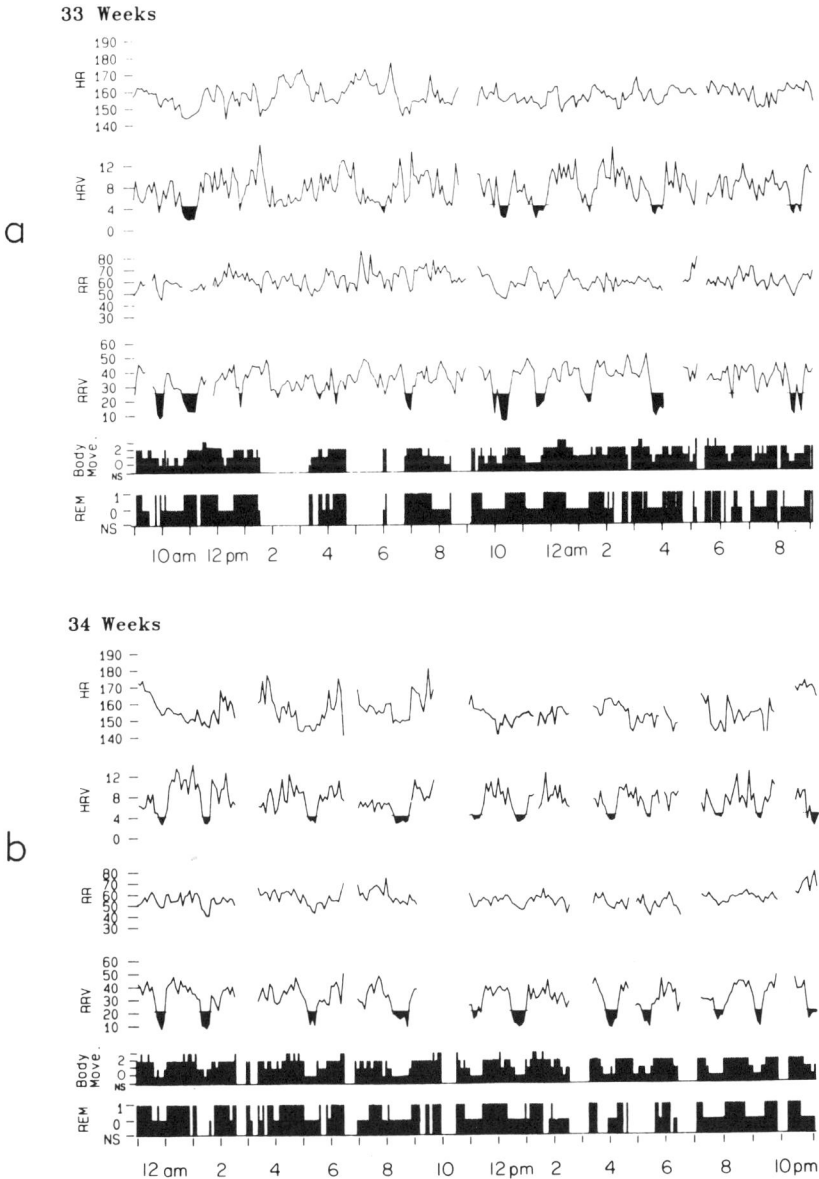

Figure 4. Twenty-four hour polygraphic tracings for one infant in study at 33 weeks' (a) and 34 weeks' (b) conceptional age, showing heart rate (HR), heart rate variability (HRV), respiratory rate (RR), respiratory rate variability (RRV), body movement, and eye movement (REM). Note that filled-in segments of RRV and HRV, indicating low variability, a criterion for quiet sleep, mostly occur when there are no eye movements and no or few body movements.

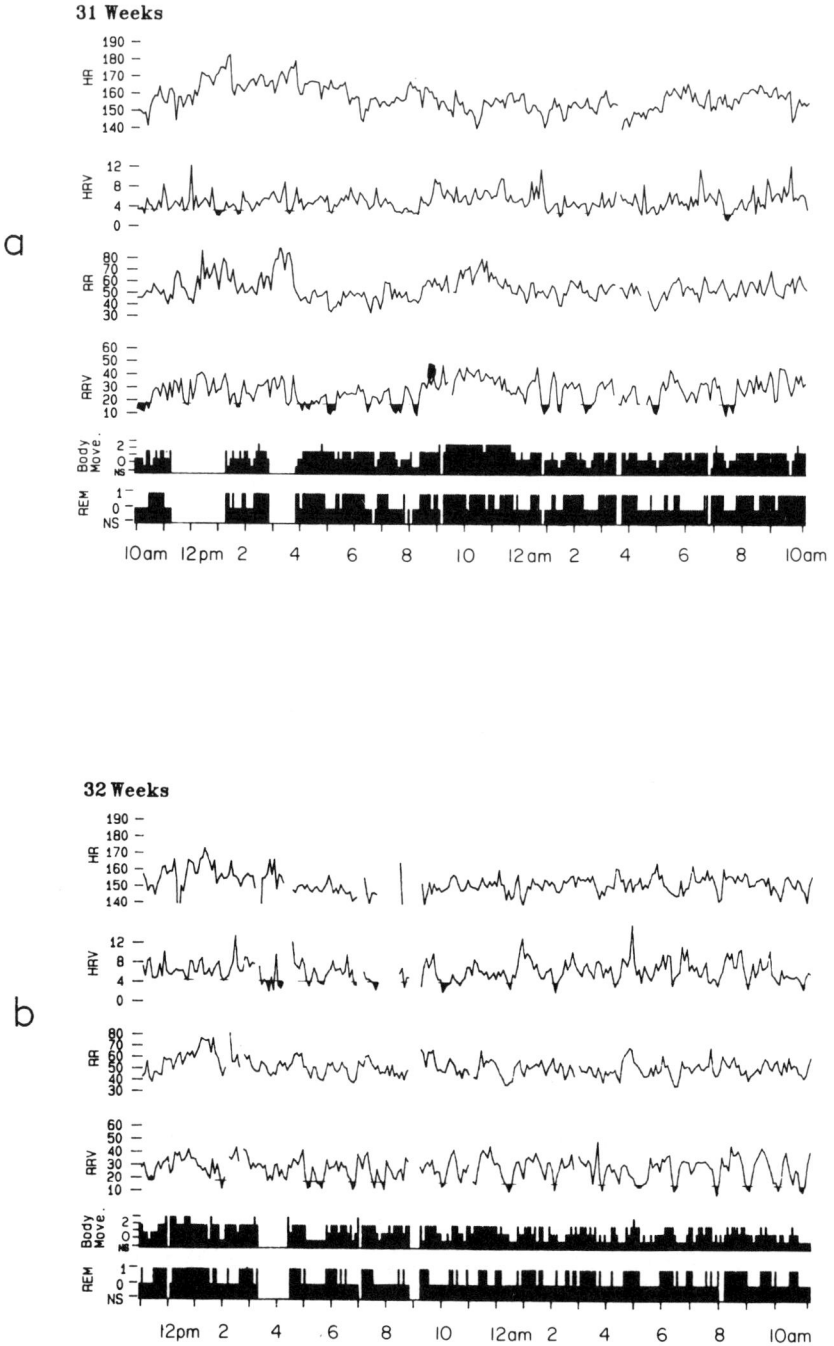

Figure 5. Twenty-four hour polygraphic tracings for a younger infant at 31
weeks' (a) and 32 weeks' (b) conceptional age. See figure 4 for
explanation of graph.

period classified as awake was between 9:00 p.m and midnight, when the infant was in almost continuous movement, had high respiratory and heart rates, and had high respiratory rate variability. This infant's sleep state profile one week later, at 32 weeks' conceptional age, does not show much better organization, consisting of 9 percent quiet sleep, 24 percent active sleep, 14 percent awake, and 53 percent indeterminate state. Although the infant was considered well at this time, during the entire week between the two recordings the infant had been under treatment that necessitated repeated medical intervention. Perhaps the infant stayed somewhat disorganized because of these intrusions.

These 24-hour profiles depict the global organization of sleep and awake states while the infant is in the NICU. Microanalytic studies were also performed on individual state parameters—respiration, heart rate, and body movement—and their interactions. These microanalyses revealed differences in the physiological organization between the two subjects and sometimes between the different ages. Compared with the younger, sicker infant, the older and healthier infant showed: (1) a more consistent shape in the distribution from one week to the next in respiratory rate variability and heart rate variability; (2) heart rate to be more sensitive to movement; (3) a greater range in the variability of heart rate; and (4) respiratory sinus arrhythmia—the integration of heart and respiratory rates—to be more pronounced and consistent from week to week.

Conclusion

These examples illustrate the types of detailed studies of state organization that can be done on long-term polygraphic recordings and the potential of such analyses for defining more clearly the progressive organization of states and the interaction of this organization with environmental stimuli. Long-term polygraphic recordings can thus provide a backdrop of the physiological organization of the infant for viewing the effects of short-term interactions of the infant with hospital caregivers, parents, and other sources of environmental stimulation.

DISCUSSION

Jennifer Buchwald: Is there a clear definition of *preterm* that we agree upon? Does it have to do with time in the uterus? Does it have to do with the organizational state of the infant? Does it have to do with some kind of measurable parameter or is there a range, so that even some whom we would call term infants actually reflect physiological disorganization that could be related to preterm infants?

Arthur Parmelee: We use *preterm* to designate infants born at gestational ages of less than 40 weeks (*term*). Usually less than 37 weeks' gestation is stipulated. At one time we used only a weight of less than 2,500 grams as an indicator of preterm birth, but then it became clear that infants could be full-term, 40 weeks' gestational age, and have low weights. We also used the term *premature*, but then the question was, less mature than what, since the full-term infant is also not mature, and we shifted to the designation *preterm* infant. Preterm infants can, therefore, vary in gestational age at birth from 24 to 37 weeks, and they have different levels of physiological organization at each gestational and conceptional age. We use *conceptional* age to indicate gestational age plus age from birth. Thus, an infant born at 29 weeks' gestational age but recorded two weeks after birth is 31 weeks' conceptional age at the time of recording.

Jennifer Buchwald: But doesn't the gestational/conceptional age ratio also make a big difference? Is that taken into consideration in these kinds of measurements?

Arthur Parmelee: This is an important issue that I have attempted to address in other studies, and Anneliese Korner has addressed it with more sophisticated statistical studies. In our current study, however, we are using a within-subject design.

Michael Schwartz: Exactly what do you mean by a "better organized" baby?

Arthur Parmelee: Better organized, for me, is indicated when the several parameters of a state run together for extended periods of time. For example, if a child can sustain a regular heart rate, regular respirations, no eye movements, and a minimum of body movements for a durable period of time, this is considered well-organized quiet sleep. If a child can then alternate that with sustained periods of active sleep several times in a day, we would consider that child well organized. It is also true that there can be too rigid organization that can militate against survival under certain circumstances. Under certain stresses, it may be important to break down state constellations into their parts to allow for greater adaptability of each variable.

Michael Schwartz: So in a sense that definition is biased against the awake time?

Arthur Parmelee: I think it may be biased because of our interest in the importance of sleep states, particularly quiet sleep, for coping with stimulation. But that still has to be determined.

Nico Spinelli: This concept of organization makes some unspoken assumptions about the mechanisms behind it. Even if those assumptions are wrong, it's nice to have them clear, because they provide a point of departure. One way of looking at this has to do with biorhythms, which imply cyclic mechanisms—circadian and so on. Another way of looking at it has to do with homeostatic mechanisms, feedback groups which keep physiological parameters within certain ranges. In that case I look at respiration, which is a cycling phenomenon, as something which could be either completely caused by a feedback mechanism or as a cyclic mechanism under the control of the homeostatic mechanism. And finally, computer scientists talk of state as a different constellation of features, which doesn't imply anything about sectors or field or whatever. It might be cycles or not; it's just a different constellation of parameters. So for my clarity of mind, which one of these concepts is involved, or are all these involved in this definition of *organized?*

Arthur Parmelee: The concept that we are using, which may be absolutely fallacious, is an engineering concept. In quiet sleep, for example, the infant sustains, over a period of time, regular respiration, regular heart rate, and absence of movement. This requires some biofeedback controlling mechanism for each parameter and a higher order feedback loop that keeps them all in synchrony. One can also add to that EEG, a measure of cortical activity, and demand that specific EEG patterns be coincident with the other quiet sleep parameters. This adds still another level of organizational integration. The same is true for active sleep. On the other hand, a mixture of EEG patterns occurs during indeterminate states of sleep. We are attempting to study the ontogeny of the organization of each parameter of state separately and in coordination with each other as states. For the youngest preterm infants, for example, movement doesn't alter heart rate very much. As these infants mature, heart rate changes are increasingly influenced by movement. Similarly, in the youngest preterm infant, there is less locking of respiration and heart rate as measured by sinus arrhythmia, and with maturation the interaction between heart rate and respiration increases. Gradually, with maturation all the parameters of each state interact and form state constellations.

Frances Horowitz: Hawley, how many of the state observations can be made by just going in and looking at the baby for the various criteria?

Arthur Parmelee: Certainly some of them can. I think the greatest difficulty has always been that one of the best quiet sleep criteria, regular respiration, is not as easy to judge in preterm infants as in term or older infants. It is difficult to get two people to agree on what to designate as regular respirations in an infant who has mostly irregular respirations and is only sometimes less irregular. I think if we make these judgments first with direct recordings and statistically, we may learn to eyeball respiratory regularity and irregularity almost as well. This should be easiest, of course, during quiet sleep. In awake states it will be harder because of the moment-to-moment changes.

Frances Horowitz: One of the most interesting things is breaking down the awake state into its components. I think everyone knows intuitively that when you rate someone who is awake you're looking at quite different states.

Arthur Parmelee: At issue is whether one is looking at states or moments of arousal. I'm arguing at the moment that what are called awake states are not states but levels of arousal. Part of the confusion for me in the past was that I learned about sleep from Drs. Donald Lindsley and Horace Magoun, and at that time they saw sleep and awake states on a continuum of arousal. The concept changed with the studies of Kleitman, Dement, and Jouvet, who described neurophysiological state constellations. Their sleep state constellations are not considered as deeper and lighter, but as totally different one from another. Kleitman viewed different levels of wakefulness in the same way. Whether there are durable constellations of states during wakefulness on which are superimposed various levels of arousal remains to be clarified. Unfortunately, there is a tendency to designate state constellations and levels of arousal as if they were the same.

Edward Tronick: When you were using "awake," you were not necessarily meaning alert?

Arthur Parmelee: No. That's correct. Prechtl quite wisely decided not to use any of these terms but uses numbers instead. Thus he has a state number 4, which you don't have to call "awake." It's just state 4, which you can describe neurophysiologically in the way I have attempted. Specifying a state by number is helpful when you can't be sure whether it is an awake state as we know it in older infants but it is nevertheless a distinct constellation of physiological parameters that continues for a period of time.

Peter Gorski: Would you venture an opinion about the relative vulnerability or instability in active sleep states versus the transitional states? Is there more variability, physiologically, in the transitional? It seems almost by definition that active sleep might be more organized than transitional sleep, but is transitional perhaps more organized in that it is tending toward a quiet state?

Arthur Parmelee: This is a matter of much discussion, and some people refuse to use the terms *transitional* or *indeterminate* states. We now plan to use the term *indeterminate* state rather than *transitional*. Most of the time the indeterminate state periods do occur during transitions, but not always. We are really not studying transitions as organized entities. Shirake and Prechtl have studied the organization of transitions, as have other investigators. They have all been interested in whether transition periods have systematic sequences of parameter shifts to the new state. A systematic sequence has not been found as far as I know.

Frances Horowitz: Is it possible that the sequence of transition is its consequence? that for some babies transition becomes ultimately a very disorganizing experience, while other babies move through the transition and come to another state organization much more smoothly, so that in and of itself its characteristics are not critical but what it portends for the next period of time is critical?

Arthur Parmelee: I think this is an important issue, and we have not addressed it. I think we should in the future.

Jennifer Buchwald: I know that at one point you were very interested in the studies Wendell had done with anencephalic infants. I've been thinking of the way in which state is organized in these very little babies and what produces that increase in synchrony and increasing coalescence of physiological parameters. Were those anencephalic babies at all organized, or were they completely disorganized in their physiological parameters?

Arthur Parmelee: It's a little unclear, because detailed state studies weren't done, but they do organize states. The most characteristic thing about them on any measure is the stereotypic nature of all their movements, both spontaneous and elicited. Their organization seems to be so rigid it is not very adaptable to environmental changes. A system can be *too* highly organized.

BEHAVIORAL RESPONSIVITY IN PRETERM INFANTS

Cynthia Garcia Coll, Ph.D.,
Laura Emmons, B.A.,
and Laurie Anderson, R.N., M.S.

During the first year of life, preterm infants differ from full-term infants in their perceptual and information-processing abilities (see Field & Sostek, 1983). There is accumulating evidence that preterm infants might also differ in their behavioral responsiveness to both social and nonsocial stimulation. Research utilizing the Brazelton Neonatal Behavioral Assessment Scale (NBAS) with preterm and full-term infants at the time of discharge, equating for gestational age, has indicated that preterm infants score significantly lower on items requiring attention and orientation and receive lower scores on ratings of state, interactive, and motor processes (Lester et al., 1976; Goldberg, 1978; Sostek, Quinn, & Davitt, 1979). In general, preterm infants are considered to be less alert, less active, and less socially responsive than full-term infants during the neonatal period and through the first few months of life.

Several investigators, however, have documented both hypo- and hyperresponsiveness in preterm infants, depending on the intensity of the stimulus and the kind of response being measured—for example, behavioral or cardiac response (Bench & Parker, 1971; Field et al., 1979; Howard et al., 1976; Krafchuk, Tronick, & Clifton, 1983). Moreover, most studies to date have focused on group differences, considering preterm infants as a homogeneous group, not taking into consideration the type and degree of perinatal complications experienced by the infant.

Using a framework of infant temperament, the research described in this paper assesses the infant's behavioral style in terms of positive or negative affect, activity, sociability, and soothability in response to a series of visual, auditory, and tactile stimulations. The long-term goals of these studies are: (1) to extend the findings of differential patterns of responsivity in preterm infants beyond the neonatal period; (2) to relate the different types and degrees of perinatal problems to behavioral responsivity in preterm infants; (3) to examine the relationship between neonatal behavior and behavioral responsiveness at later ages; and (4) to assess the relationship between behavioral observations of responsivity and parental reports of the infant's temperament and to cardiac responses.

Effects of Intraventricular Hemorrhage on Behavior in Preterm Infants

In the first study, our objective was to assess the effects of prematurity and differing degrees of intraventricular hemorrhage on behavioral responsivity at three months corrected age.

Intraventricular hemorrhage (IVH) has been identified as the most common central nervous system autopsy lesion found in premature infants (Towbin, 1970). More recently, with the development of cranial ultrasound and computerized axial tomography (CAT), IVH has been found in 30 to 50 percent of low-birthweight infant survivors (Papile et al., 1978; Ahmann et al., 1980). A recent study by Papile and her colleagues, which utilized her scoring system for grading cerebral IVH into Grades I, II, III, and IV, found a significant relationship between severity of hemorrhage and severity of neurological handicap (Papile, Munsick-Bruno, & Schaefer, 1983).

For the study we recruited full-term infants without major prenatal or perinatal complications. We also recruited preterm infants who were less than 1,750 grams and 34 weeks' gestational age at birth. In the latter group, cranial ultrasounds were performed at two, seven, and fourteen days of life. The infants were classified as not having a hemorrhage, having an isolated germinal matrix hemorrhage (Grade I), having an accompanied IVH with no ventricular dilatation (Grade II), having an IVH with ventricular dilatation (Grade III), or having an IVH with ventricular dilatation and seepage into the white matter (Grade IV).

The NBAS (Brazelton, 1973) was administered to the full-term infants within two days after birth and to the preterm infants at 40 weeks' conceptional age. The NBAS for both full-term and preterm infants was scored, using an established system, into seven clusters: habituation, orientation, motor, state range, state regulation, autonomic stability, and reflexes (Lester, Als, & Brazelton, 1982). At three to four months (corrected age for the preterms) the ICQ (Bates et al., 1979) was given to the mothers to fill out and was scored into four scores: fussy-difficult, unadaptable, dull, and unpredictable.

Behavioral responsivity was also assessed at three to four months for both full-term and preterm infants, using fifteen visual, auditory, and tactile stimuli, such as dangling a brightly colored toy, cuddling, brushing the infant's hair, ringing a bell, and presenting an overwhelming toy. The responses were scored for positive or negative affect, sociability, soothability, and overall activity.

The statistical analysis of the seven Brazelton NBAS clusters showed group differences in four clusters: orientation, state range, state regulation, and deviant reflexes. Preterm infants with Grade III-IV IVH had significantly lower orientation scores than full-term controls or preterm infants with no IVH or with Grade I-II. On state range, the presence of hemorrhage, regardless of grade, seems to affect adversely the infant's range of state. Lower scores in state regulation and a greater number of deviant reflexes are associated with prematurity and not necessarily with the presence or degree of IVH. Thus, depending on the dimension of neonatal behavior examined, effects of prematurity or of IVH can be detected even at 40 weeks' conceptional age.

In the behavioral responsivity scores at three months, there were significant differences for the positive, sociability, soothability, and overall activity scores. Preterm infants, regardless of presence or degree of intraventricular hemorrhage, were less positive and less active than full-term controls. In addition, preterm infants with a Grade I-II IVH were less sociable and less soothable as a group than full-term infants.

We also examined the relationship between behavioral responsivity and the maternal ratings on the Bates ICQ. For the preterm infants as a group, higher scores on the Bates dimensions of fussy-difficult and unadaptable were related to lower positive scores, higher negative scores, less sociability, and less soothability. Thus, our behavioral observations are moderately related to maternal perceptions of the infant's temperament, which can have implications for the developing mother-infant interaction (Milliones, 1978).

Cardiac Responses and Behavioral Responsivity

A second study is now underway to reassess the impact of prematurity and perinatal complications on behavioral responsivity. As part of this study, we will assess the relationship of behavior to concurrent measures of cardiac reactivity. Previous studies (for example, Field et al., 1979) have suggested that cardiac changes in preterm infants show a defensive pattern of responsivity not necessarily observed in behavioral responses.

We have analyzed the heart rate and heart rate variability of eight infants during the presentation of each stimulus on the behavioral responsivity assessment. Preterm and full-term infants had similar cardiac responses during the initial face-to-face stimulus, but then preterm infants tended to have higher heart rates than full-term infants in response to cuddling and caretaking activities and to an auditory stimulus. Paradoxically, to more intense (such as a jack-in-the-box) or discrepant stimulation (masks), their heart rates decreased.

Conclusions

It is clear that both prematurity and the type and degree of perinatal complication affect behavioral responsivity. The lower levels of sociability and soothability shown by preterm infants can be considered to be due to some stress to the central nervous system. Marked individual differences are observed within preterm groups, however, and stimulation should therefore be geared to the individual infant's level of responsivity.

DISCUSSION

Barry Nurcombe: You are suggesting that the difference between the Grade III-IVs and the Grade I-IIs is that the former are relatively unreactive or unresponsive, their reactions are dampened. Is that a conjecture, or is it an observation?

Cynthia Garcia Coll: There is no statistical difference between Grade I-II and Grade III-IV in most of the behavioral responsivity measures at three to four months of age. My clinical impression, however, is that these babies are reacting less.

Barry Nurcombe: Did you actually see that unreactivity, or nonreactivity? What are the indices of unreactivity?

Cynthia Garcia Coll: With some of these children, there's no protest to anything, whatever you do. You can put the hat on, turn them around—there's never any irritability. We've seen that when we do behavioral assessments with some of the preemies during the perinatal period. The group that stands out is the Grade I-II. For some reason or other those children are more negative and more difficult to soothe. The whole notion that preemies are more negative and unsoothable might be coming from that group and not necessarily from the other two.

Frances Horowitz: I'm wondering about the large variability in your preterm group, and whether some of what you're getting is an artifact of that variability. If you could find a way to break down the three preterm groups by pulling out some babies who on one of the measures are closer to your term group, and then those who are very variable, you might get a more regular relationship between neonatal behavior and temperament.

Cynthia Garcia Coll: Variability based on behavior or on heart rate?

Frances Horowitz: That would be the question. I think I'd look at the distributions and then see if there's some way to divide the preterm groups that might show you some more consistent patterns.

Barry Nurcombe: My understanding is that when the ventricles are enlarged or the hemorrhage seeps into the white matter beyond the basal ganglia, then that causes neurological damage—low IQ, I think, in at least one study.

Cynthia Garcia Coll: Yes, there are a couple of studies by Papile and other investigators who have looked at Grades III and IV and their relationship to neurological damage. Especially with Grade IV it is very high. We're following these children through the first three years of life, and we're finding that it's only around two-thirds of the Grade IVs that have some major neurological damage.

Nico Spinelli: How do you detect bleeding that produces no ventricular dilatation when reading ultrasounds? What do you see?

Cynthia Garcia Coll: You see opacity in the ventricles.

Nico Spinelli: Many years ago Feldman demonstrated that extremely small amounts of substances injected in the ventricular fluid of healthy animals had tremendously large behavioral effects. So from that point of view, when you get larger amounts you may have unpredictable effects.

Cynthia Garcia Coll: That's my impression in the Grade III-IV bleeds.

Nico Spinelli: On the other hand, with the Grade I-II reaction, you may have just small amounts of blood and related materials that might have stimulating effects.

Jennifer Buchwald: Is it possible to do any kind of CAT scan on these babies, so that you have an idea where the hemorrhage is?

Robert Isaacson: I was going to ask these same sorts of questions. It's a mystery to me how you could be sure of what you're seeing in the ultrasound. And it should be known, I would think, which particular areas are being affected. I'm not sure a CAT scan would do it. PET scans and/or NMR might be better.

If you cannot use imaging methods, you might think of various pharmacologic challenges. Even small amounts of norepinephrine, epinephrine, or various other pharmacologic agents might give you some hint as to where the dysfunction is located. For example, if you give a small dose of clonidine to an animal with damage restricted to the neocortex, it will produce a drop of three or four degrees in temperature. If the animal doesn't have neocortical damage, the drop will be only about one degree. Tests like this could give a clear indication of the nature of the damage.

Jennifer Buchwald: Why isn't it possible to use either a CAT scan or nucleomagnetic resonance to get a real definition of what's going on?

Arthur Parmelee: These studies are being done. The issues are logistic, and so far such studies, while very revealing, are not often combined with behavioral studies. Sonography is helpful because it can be done serially. The real issue is when a hemorrhage starts and when it ends and how quickly it resolves. A great many hemorrhages resolve without any apparent damage to the brain. Unless you follow their progress with sonography you don't know when you would get your most revealing CAT scan, NMR, or PET scan. These pieces of the information are now being gradually brought together. There are some lesions being found, particularly those described as leucomalacia, that are significantly related to abnormal outcomes. I think eventually we will know when and where to look. At this point most often we focus on the behavior and sonography, waiting for the results of more complex approaches being done by a number of pediatric neurologists.

Berry Brazelton: Cindy, you're putting your finger on something I see clinically all the time with premature infants after they come out of the preemie nursery. I think this kind of hypersensitivity comes from an area that's damaged and is trying to repair itself. You get a major hypersensitivity around that area, but then you get a spread to the whole brain. I think you're seeing that in your Grade I-II. And this capacity to shut down, which is intact and becomes necessary with the more massive intrusions that you do at the end, is something that mothers have to deal with all the time with their preemies for quite a while after discharge. Whether it's induced by the kind of environments we have them in or recovery from the insult, I don't think we have any idea.

Cynthia Garcia Coll: I'm very interested to see if our findings replicate with a larger sample: the notion that in the preterm versus the full-term the heart rate goes down as stimulation goes up—the opposite of what we would expect. It also ties up with some of Tronick's previous work in what you might call the paradoxical reaction. Some preterm infants seem unreactive, but then all of a sudden they are crying, out of control. Then there is nothing that will console them. So initially they seem unresponsive, and after a certain level of stimulation they are over-responsive.

Berry Brazelton: At a medical level, hemorrhage Grade I-II may be unimportant to us, but certainly it may be important to parents, because some of the babies they take home are very disordered and very distressed.

Cynthia Garcia Coll: I think that that's the importance of this work. The general attitude is that infants with Grade I-II IVH don't have major neurological problems, so we don't have to worry about them. And what I am saying is that there are some behavioral consequences to that insult that might be very important for parents, specifically within the first six months of life.

Edward Tronick: I think that simply focusing on the bleed as characterizing these infants leaves out the fact that the physiology may be more compromised in the Grade IV infants. These are infants who might be characterized as recovering from severe illness with or without attendant brain damage. Hyperreactivity and hyposensitivities and those other dimensions can grow out of physiology or they can grow out of stress or brain damage or combinations of all these factors.

Cynthia Garcia Coll: Right. For the Grade I-II infants, hospitalization days were very high. It might be that the Grade I-II is just a marker for other perinatal events.

BEHAVIORAL ORGANIZATION OF THE NEWBORN PRETERM INFANT: APATHETIC ORGANIZATION MAY NOT BE ABNORMAL

Edward Tronick, Ph.D.,
Kathleen B. Scanlon, M.S.N.,
and John W. Scanlon, M.D.

There are few studies of the behavior of extremely preterm infants during the newborn period. Typically studies have employed behavioral examinations designed for full-term infants, with or without modifications in content, administering them to preterm infants at term conceptional age or at discharge from the hospital. Two conditions accounted for this situation. First, it was difficult if not impossible to maintain homeostasis in an extremely small or ill infant during a behavioral examination. Second, no appropriate behavioral assessment technique was available for use with newly born preterms.

Both of these conditions have changed. Standard procedures and technology now make it possible to maintain homeostasis during a behavioral examination, and modifications of the Brazelton (1973) full-term examination (NBAS) have been developed to study the ontogeny of behavior in the preterm infant, starting prior to term. These modified examinations are the Assessment of Preterm Infant Behavior (A.P.I.B., Als et al., 1982) and its forerunner, the Brazelton Premature Scale (PREMIE, Als, Tronick, & Brazelton, 1978; Scanlon, Scanlon, & Tronick, 1984; Sell, Luick, & Poisson, 1980). These assessments now permit us to study interactions between postconceptional maturation, serious disruptions in physiological homeostasis, and neurodevelopmental ontogeny and to use such studies to guide interventions.

This paper describes the behavioral organization and its change in relation to physiological and clinical variables in a group of very low birthweight (VLBW) infants. These infants represent a clinical population of infants experiencing and recovering from acute cardiorespiratory illness. We used the PREMIE, an examination designed for use with a wide range of gestational ages (27 to 35 weeks). Examinations began one week after birth and were obtained serially during the initial recovery period of the infants.

Methods

The study included 45 infants with birthweights between 750 and 1,500 grams. They ranged in gestational age from 26 to 34 weeks.

Many infants were receiving oxygen or other ventilatory support, as well as intravenous therapy, heart and respiratory rate monitoring, and/or $TcPO_2$ monitoring. These infants were examined on heated tables or in isolettes. Many rest periods were provided during testing on the basis of trends in clinical signs and monitoring data, and examination was terminated if an infant did not recover spontaneously within ten seconds from an episode of tachypnea, bradycardia, tachycardia, or hypoxemia. Infants requiring ventilatory support were manipulated and handled as little as possible, and the number and sequence of items administered was modified.

For the purposes of this study, the infants' scores on the PREMIE were recorded twice. Time 1 was on average seven days after birth, and Time 2 was on average 21 days after birth. Their subscores and total (overall) scores on these examinations were correlated with clinical data (such, as cord pH, high and low pO2, low systolic pressure, peak bilirubin level, and the duration of mechanical ventilation, oxygen exposure, and theophylline therapy) as well as with birth demographic factors (such as gestational age, birthweight, birth length, birth head circumference, and Apgar scores).

Correlations Among Birth Demographics, Physiological Variables, and PREMIE Scores

As is done with the NBAS, the individual scores on the PREMIE are grouped in typology sum scores that summarize the infant's performance in different functional domains (e.g., orientation or motor performance). These sum scores were found to be strongly interrelated, suggesting that these infants have few domains of differentiated performance available to them.

Detailed descriptive data and correlations are reported elsewhere (Tronick, Scanlon, & Scanlon, in press). At seven days of age, the descriptors of perinatal asphyxia, such as cord pH, accounted for significant variance on the PREMIE. Lowest recorded pO2 and duration of oxygen exposure also emerged as important influences on behavior. The results indicate that gestational age, birthweight, and Apgar scores are poor predictors of behavior in these infants at this time. Thus indices of acute illness rather than indices of immaturity per se were most closely related to behavior.

This observation appears to strengthen the argument that birth circumstances amenable to medical intervention may have a greater influence on neonatal behavior in these infants than does maturity itself. This idea is concordant with the clinically popular view that perinatal asphyxia and the quality of resuscitative efforts influence the severity and course of many acute neonatal illnesses.

Observations on the second examination (day 21) reveal a stronger emerging influence of maturational processes along with an abatement of the previously strong effects of acute birth factors, such as asphyxia. Gestational age and birthweight exhibit higher correlations with behavior scores on this examination. Length and head circumference at birth similarly reveal stronger correlations. The correlation of cord pH and behavior is less significant than on the first examination. By 21 days of age, with some recovery from acute events, behavior begins to reflect more strongly neurological maturational processes and clinical course.

Nutritional adequacy appears to be increasingly important for behavioral functioning, as suggested by correlations between weight at the time of the examination and the total PREMIE score at Time 2. Unfortunately, there is little data on specific nutritional requirements for VLBW babies at various times after birth. The recommendations for proper growth trajectories for such babies are controversial. On an empirical basis, the influence of nutrition on postnatal neurobehavioral development appears great.

Discussion of Behavioral Data and Conclusions

At Time 1, these VLBW babies are extremely poorly organized in all domains of behavior functioning. Their behavior improves at Time 2, but it is still poor. There is significant stability in their performance over this time.

This behavioral organization can be classified as relatively abnormal by criteria based on the full-term or even the healthy preterm infant (Amiel-Tison, 1968; Prechtl, 1968; Tronick & Brazelton, 1975; Drillien, 1974). But we do not really know what is abnormal for these infants. Normal development typically proceeds from undifferentiated to differentiated and from unintegrated to integrated. This is the pattern seen with these infants, and it is not surprising that these extremely immature and ill infants are diffusely organized, lacking in specificity, and without integrated functioning, especially at Time 1. These infants do not yet evidence differentiated dimensions of behavior but rather show a global and diffuse organization. In fact it was found that a single summary measure of behavioral performance was as strongly related to physiological and clinical variables as were any of the different typology sum scores.

At Time 1 these infants are physiologically unstable, dependent for survival on the entire therapeutic repertoire of the modern neonatologist. At Time 2 maintenance of physiologic stability, though much less problematic, still requires parenteral fluids and nutrition, external support from heat sources, and often enriched oxygen environments. Even the physiologically most stable of these infants require monitoring of their functions and occasional interventions. Their behavior is related to their physiologic status. Initially such potentially life-threatening factors as acidosis and severe respiratory disease are most strongly related to behavior. By Time 2 other, less acute conditions such as weight change and peak bilirubin level are most strongly related. The infants' behavior reflects these homeostatic demands, the transition to this less acute condition, and the emergence of maturational forces initially masked by their acute physiologic condition.

At Time 1 these infants are in sleep states most of the time. They seldom move into alert states, and they do not move into states of crying even when disturbed. They make few state changes. They are not irritable, and responsiveness is difficult to elicit. When they are brought to a state of alertness, often by a good deal of examiner effort, its duration is short and the infants' orientation is poor. Moreover, alertness is accompanied by multiple signs of stress. The shift back to sleep comes quickly and is abrupt. At Time 2 the infants have a wider range of states, but their predominant state is still sleep. The duration of alertness has increased, and their specific orientation capacities are improved. Alertness remains difficult to elicit, however, and is accompanied by signs of stress. Habituation performance has not changed from Time 1 in any meaningful way. Motorically, they are only slightly more active at Time 2 than at Time 1.

The infants' behavioral organization may be interpreted as apathetic and therefore "abnormal." An alternative interpretation, however, is that by being asleep, inactive, and unresponsive they conserve energy and utilize these savings of energy to achieve and maintain homeostasis. Thus their behavioral organization can be seen as a protective mechanism that aids recovery, a normal behavioral organization for this type of infant. Moreover, it functions as a communication to a caregiver to reduce the amount of stimulation the infant is exposed to and to support the infant's protective organization.

This protective apathy has several implications for the assessment and care of these infants. Assessment needs to focus on the functional task of the infant, who is primarily faced with trying to achieve homeostasis. Initially assessment should focus on the changeover from the influence of acute physiologic events to the influence of more chronic conditions on behavior. Certainly this is what medical management should focus upon. If the interpretation offered above is correct, behavioral assessment might focus upon an infant's ability to remain unresponsive and inactive to maintain this protective apathy, rather than to become alert.

As homeostatic stability is achieved, assessment should track the emergence of differentiated states of sleep, alertness, and crying, along with an increase in activity and responsiveness. Then with the emergence of clearly bounded states, assessment could focus on their integration, the transitions among them, and their lability. Assessment could now also be made of the specific orientation capacities, habituation, and motor performances within states.

This view of initial assessment and of a protective apathetic state fits with Brazelton's (1975) hypothesis that sleep states can be used effectively by the infant to defend himself against disturbing stimuli prior to the development of the ability to habituate. It also fits to more classic ideas on the stimulus barrier as a protective mechanism aiding the infant in maintaining self-regulation (Spitz, 1965; Freud, 1920; Emde & Robinson, 1976). Overall it supports Tronick's formulation of the paradoxical reactivity hypothesis, in which preterm infants are viewed as having a high stimulus threshold and a low defensive reaction threshold, making them generally appear hyporesponsive except when a stimulus is strong enough to cross the stimulus threshold, when they appear hyperreactive. The results certainly are not compatible with views that emphasize the assessment of highly specific functions in these infants.

With hindsight, the examination used in this study, devoting as it did so much energy to characterizing the details of the infant's performance, seems inappropriate. It might be better to develop an assessment instrument graded for an infant's level of development and degree of illness or to impose a developmental illness matrix on the assessment used for these types of studies.

It is clear that assessment needs to be made repeatedly during this period. It is the infant's progress through these tasks that will indicate the infant's capacity to recover (Brazelton, 1978; Lester, 1983). This tracking of recovery is especially critical with these infants, because much of their performance looks abnormal. It is our view that only an infant's ability to accomplish one task and to begin the next one can distinguish him or her from those infants who will not recover.

The infants in this study can be described as unavailable to stimulation and easily stressed by it. They do not seem able to use stimulation to help themselves get organized, as does the full-term infant. Certainly any extra stimulation seems uncalled for. Indeed, it seems reasonable to argue that a reduction in input would serve them best and that when stimulation is introduced it should be specifically fitted to the development task of the infant at that time.

What should be our expectations about parental involvement with these infants? The infants in this study demonstrated little capacity to play their role in interaction with their caregivers. Even a highly skilled and experienced examiner had difficulty in interacting with these infants. How much greater might be the difficulties for a parent who has just experienced a series of psychological and physiological stresses? Will the parent simply experience one more failure by trying to interact with an unresponsive child? But the implication is not that parents should be excluded from the nursery, but that practitioners should rethink the demands they place on parents.

A principle that might be used to guide this reevaluation is that practices should support the development of maternal and paternal self-esteem. Shea and Tronick (in press) found that mothers with higher self-esteem interacted more appropriately with their sick and well infants. With infants such as those described in this paper, practices helpful to parental feelings of effectiveness might be graded to fit the behavior of the infant. Initially, contact with the infant could emphasize the increasing physiological stability and growth of the infant. Interaction with the infant might be limited and determined by the parents. Then as the infant's responsiveness improved, interaction might be encouraged. Such an approach would aid both the parents and the infant.

DISCUSSION

Peter Gorski: You seem to be saying that the preterm infant through its behavior is acting as a communicator. I always wonder if we're stretching the concept of communication a little bit, whether it may not be that the infant presents some cues that we respond to and over time we teach the infant that there is a replication of results and that he or she can effectively begin to communicate a need or a stage or an affect.

Edward Tronick: I think that point is well taken. One definition of communication is that it's in the receiver, not in the sender. With that definition, then certainly we can make use of those kinds of communications. I certainly don't mean to imply communication in the way we use the word later in development. But one can take the view that these behaviors are part of an involved communication system, but one that was never designed for the preterm infant. Nonetheless the communications that the preterm is using may be ones that the full-term and older child uses, so that indeed we are sensitive to them. Maybe they have some behaviors that we don't know about yet, that we're not sensitive to but that also would be useful as communications.

All I mean is that we must watch these infants very carefully, to see what it is that they're trying to do. You don't see them quietly looking around, seeking out stimulation. You don't see them responding with relaxed facial expressions to the approach of the examiner, and you don't see them turning to the examiner with eyes open and relaxed faces when you give them auditory stimulation. What you see are signs of stress, or what can be seen as conveying the message that "I'm getting unregulated and need to be left alone." And I think we can respond to that.

Kathryn Barnard: This infant communication theory has been of interest to me. We've looked at infant activity over time with 24-hour time lapse video recording and also recorded their caregiving intervention. One caregiving intervention that declines over time is touching and stroking. I've often wondered, do infants put out subtle messages that it is wrong to touch them? There is historically a very strong dogma about handling the baby as little as possible, and I think that we need more investigation of these very low-level communications that are giving caregivers these kinds of signals. I think they have developed for a reason.

Berry Brazelton: That's what's so interesting about what you might call the intuitive aspect that Cindy brought up. You know, we really need a better goal-oriented way of classifying babies than just preterm and full-term. And the preterm babies take a lot longer to get out of the phase of needing to defend themselves in order to organize internally. To think that they might start looking before they are well enough organized to manage that kind of demand is, I guess, where we're going wrong in comparing them, and where we certainly might go wrong in any kind of stimulation program.

Edward Tronick: I think you used the word *convalescence*. One of the models I use with my students in teaching them high-risk assessment is a model of convalescence of these infants. I use the analogy of adults who suffer severe illnesses and the length of time it takes them to recover. I think some of the clinical pediatric literature is also conceptualizing these infants more in terms of their illness than in terms of preterm or full-term.

Cynthia Garcia Coll: How long should we think about the premature infant as convalescing from this illness? Is it six or eight months? Is it for a year? What are we talking about? Two years?

Berry Brazelton: When mothers ask me now, I say seven years.

Arthur Parmelee: The more practical issue is how long intervention programs should be. Are three months enough, or four months, or six months? It would appear that one year may be too short a time. In the end, what is feasible in terms of time, money, and energy may be the deciding factor.

Edward Tronick: But I think if you take the model of convalescence, then you have to raise questions about what it is that the system does during convalescence that maintains the normal rate of development of systems such as the brain. Because of the work I do in Peru, I've always wondered about torpor states. There's interesting work on the bat, of all things. A pregnant bat can go into torpor, and the rate of development of the fetus during pregnancy slows down. Then, when the torpor is ended, pregnancy is "resumed" wherever it was. So there's no average gestational age for some species of bats. Well, if you have an organism—let us say, the Peruvian infant sleeping all the time, is the rate of development modified so that it's actually slowed down? Could that occur, say, to the brain? to the rest of the body? We know that for the body there's catch-up growth. You can slow the rate down, and if the delay is not too great, you can get back on course. If we modified state in a certain way, could you slow down some of those rate parameters for other organ systems including behavior without damaging the systems?

Berry Brazelton: Lombroso did some EEG work with prematures. He found that the EEG in sleep didn't make any progress while they were sick. It was only when they were recovering that they began to make progress, and then they had a catch-up program.

Michael Schwartz: In the visual deprivation literature there are some studies suggesting that cats have a critical period when deprivation effects can change the physiology of the system. If you keep a cat in the dark for a prolonged period of time and then you come back after a year or so and deprive it unilaterally, for instance, you get the same type of effect as you would have if you had done the deprivation within the critical period, as if you prolonged that critical period by shutting down the system totally during the normal critical period.

Nico Spinelli: The convalescence model has some interesting implications. At one time doctors used to keep a patient with even a simple appendectomy in bed for several weeks, and then the patient was out of commission for months and months. Now they kick them out of bed almost immediately. So I see two models in our discussion. One model is "Leave me alone, I'm trying to set up my inner world interface," in which case, you want to leave them alone. The other model has to do with convalescing from an illness, in which case you really want to challenge them, so that they recover as fast as possible. These two points of view, I think, have very different implications for intervention.

Edward Tronick: Yes, I think this is the same thing as the stress/nonstress kind of model. Do we want them to have no episodes of anything? Or is it okay to have some stressful episodes?

Kathryn Barnard: I've often noticed that before a baby will come to a nice interactive state of quiet alert, you have to take him through an irritable, disorganized period. There seems to be a kind of disorganization that is necessary to break through before you can get the consolidation. And if you keep putting that off and not giving the child the experience of getting through some of that disorganization, you keep putting off this optimal state for interaction.

Tiffany Field: I wonder how much the initial handling of the baby is associated by the baby with aversive procedures, so that when you first approach the baby to do any kind of stimulation, there might be a conditioned association.

Craig Ramey: I think that to the degree that we are imposing stimulation that is not contingent upon what the child is doing, we may be driving arousal level up very quickly. To the extent that the child can regulate the intensity of the stimulation, it might be almost impossible for the child to overstimulate himself. In our attempt to engage the child, however, we are frequently so overpowering that we don't get a very good match between the level of the cue being given, if it is a cue, and the level of our response. One of the things we need to work on is how the child can regulate the level of input that he or she receives.

Edward Tronick: I think you are absolutely right. And with infants this young and this ill, really skillful examiners are so good at reading cues that they get optimal performances out of the infant. Because of their experience, these examiners are able to read very subtle signs and titrate their behavior closely to the infant signals. But even in that situation, there is so little indication of availability to input that the titration is probably supporting the infant's organization rather than trying to bring out other things. And personally, I think it might be better to wait until the infant begins to show some initiative spontaneously before trying to elicit certain responses. And that runs into the problem of when you start to challenge.

Craig Ramey: Evelyn Thoman has some recent data that support that notion. She seems to offer a model that would take us beyond a primitive stimulation model, in which stimulation is viewed as something that is imposed upon the child, to a model that emphasizes reciprocity and synchrony between external and internal stimulation.

BEHAVIORAL AND PSYCHOPHYSIOLOGICAL ASSESSMENT OF THE PRETERM INFANT

Barry M. Lester, Ph.D.

Popular notions of brain plasticity have been used to support behavioral assessment and early intervention with preterm infants. The rationale is that if interventions are started early, at a time when the nervous system is most susceptible to change, potential developmental deficits can be lessened or prevented. But do we know the parameters of appropriate stimulation for preterm infants or the mechanisms by which preterm infants respond to stimulation?

This paper summarizes some findings from two longitudinal studies with preterm infants. In the first study, behavioral assessment during the neonatal period was used to predict later developmental outcome. Some surprising results suggest that what appear to be optimal behavioral responses were associated with nonoptimal outcome. In the second study, psychophysiological measures of EKG and respiration were used in an attempt to understand some of the possible mechanisms by which preterm infants respond to stimulation.

Early Attention and Later Developmental Outcome

In 1978 a group under the direction of T. Berry Brazelton started a longitudinal study of the development of preterm and term infants, with several objectives: (1) to determine the long-term predictive value of repeated scores on the Neonatal Behavioral Assessment Scale (NBAS); (2) to provide a detailed description of the early behavioral development of the preterm infant; and (3) to develop additional behavioral scales that could account for some of the characteristic behaviors of preterm infants.

One of our hypotheses was that the infant's ability to track visual and auditory stimuli while in an awake and alert state, as a measure of ability to process input from the environment, would predict positive developmental outcome. On the NBAS, the orientation cluster provides a summary score of these attentional behaviors.

Longitudinal studies are full of surprises, and ours was no exception. We tested twenty term and twenty preterm infants on the NBAS at term and term-corrected age for preterm group and two and four weeks later, or at 40, 42, and 44 weeks' post-conceptional age. When we plotted the NBAS orientation cluster scores for the preterm infants and compared them with developmental outcome on the Bayley Scales at 18 months of age, we made a rather disturbing discovery. The only three infants whose orientation scores were *above* the mean for the group of preterm infants on all three tests were the only three infants with scores below 85 on the Bayley Mental Development Index (MDI).

Our first hypothesis was that the orientation scores might not accurately reflect the quality of attention in preterm infants. There were several preterm infants in the study who showed an exaggerated, intense, or hyperalert quality that clinically we find disturbing. Fortunately we had videotaped the examinations and were able to review the tapes of the infants in question.

Quite the opposite from hyperalert, these three infants showed, if anything, a somewhat dull, flat quality of alertness. At times their following responses seemed smooth and fluid. Their muscle tone was relaxed, somewhat hypotonic, and they had long periods of alertness during which they were responsive to the orientation maneuvers. In retrospect, however, we could see that they lacked the brightness and facial participation that we associate with optimal performance. We were also struck by the amount of stage setting that the examiner had to provide in order to elicit the responses. Especially at the 40-week examination, it was only with the most careful handling, in which the examiner provided substantial aids to maintain the infant in a quiet alert state, that orientation responses could be elicited. When we examined the other NBAS cluster scores on these infants, the one cluster in which they tended to score lower than the other preterm infants was regulation of state, a measure of how the infant responds when aroused, and of the ability to respond to environmental input.

Another hypothesis that might explain these findings relates to the infant's ability to regulate input from the environment. If we assume that there are mechanisms in the nervous system that control the intake of stimuli from the environment and that the infant's ability to reject stimuli could serve to protect the nervous system from too much stimulation, it follows that the inability to reject stimulation, particularly when the nervous system is undergoing rapid growth and is recovering from the trauma of prematurity, could have adverse effects on development. It is possible that the "superior" orientation abilities of these three infants was masking an inability to regulate input from the environment.

Cardiorespiratory Activity and Later Outcome

In the second study, we decided to record physiological activity (EKG and respiration) during the administration of the NBAS. Since the elicitation of alert states and attentional responses is part of the NBAS, the examination can be used to study the relationship between attention and physiological activity. By this means we hoped to come to a better understanding of the mechanisms of the nervous system that mediate the infant's information-processing ability.

We therefore developed a recording system using FM telemetry and videotape. The infant's behavior is videotaped and the physiological activity appears as a moving strip chart at the bottom of the videotape. The examiner is able to interact with the recording system through computer interface and select segments of infant behavior for physiological analysis.

Variations in heart rate are measured using spectral analysis and the cardiac orienting response. Spectral analysis is a method for quantifying variability or periodic fluctuations in heart rate. Periodicities or rhythms at certain frequencies in heart rate are mediated by physiological systems that are important for infant attention (Porges, McCabe, & Yongue, 1982; Richards, 1987). There is a significant body of literature relating heart rate to cognitive processing in adults and information processing in older infants and children (Berg &

Berg, 1987; Graham & Clifton, 1966). Heart rate deceleration is a component of the orienting response (stimulus intake), and heart rate acceleration is a component of the defensive response (stimulus rejection). With neonates, the cardiac orienting response has been more difficult to demonstrate, seeming to depend on such factors as the nature of the stimulus, the modality of the stimulus, and the state of the infant.

The subjects for this study were ten preterm and ten term infants, all healthy and appropriate weight for gestational age. The NBAS was administered to the term infants on the third day of life and to the preterm infants at 40 weeks' conceptional age. Leads from the EKG electrodes placed on the infant's chest were plugged into a portable transmitter in the experimenter's pocket, enabling the experimenter to pick up and hold the infant and elicit the behavioral responses of the NBAS.

Of particular interest were behavioral episodes when the infant was in a quiet alert state and responding to visual and auditory stimulation. On the NBAS, following a state of quiet alertness, the infant, lying on his back, is presented a series of stimuli: animate (face, voice and face, and voice of the experimenter) and inanimate (red ball and rattle). The stimuli are presented on either side of the infant's head and in a side-to-side trajectory across the infant's field of vision, to determine the infant's ability of orient to and follow the stimulus. This is called the orientation sequence.

For this study, a segment of tape was defined including the last twenty seconds of quiet alertness prior to the introduction of orientation items and the first twenty seconds of the orientation sequence. These segments enabled us to compare changes in EKG from baseline quiet alert state to the state of response during the orientation sequence.

At nine months of age (corrected for the preterm infants) a developmental follow-up was conducted, using the Bayley Scales of Infant Development. The preliminary results from this study showed statistically significant differences between term and preterm infants on the heart-rate measures during the NBAS. Term infants showed clear evidence of the cardiac orienting response while tracking the stimulus, whereas preterm infants showed no change in heart rate when they were presented with the stimulus. Spectral analysis of the heart rate showed an increase in rhythmic activity during the attentional responsivity for the term infants but not the preterm infants.

One could interpret these findings as evidence that preterm infants are less able than term infants to attend to and process information from the environment. This could imply that preterm infants have an attentional deficit. An alternative explanation, and one more consonant with our clinical experience, has to do with the notion of threshold of responsivity. Preterm infants are often described as easily overwhelmed by stimulation. It has been suggested that they may have a lower threshold for responding to stimulation because the homeostatic mechanisms of the preterm infant are more easily overwhelmed by excessive or inappropriate stimulation. If preterm infants do have a lower threshold for stimulation than term infants, stimulation at this lower threshold could produce a response in the nervous system that prevents the infant from attending to potentially overwhelming and dangerous stimulation. Rather than a *deficit* in information processing, this interpretation could suggest an *adaptive* response in which stimulation at this lower threshold produces a central or sympathetic nervous system response that protects the infant from stimulus overload.

One implication of this hypothesis is that the inability of the nervous system to respond in this protective fashion could leave the infant at the mercy of too much stimulation. We wonder if this may not have been the case with the three infants discussed in the first study. Their higher scores may have indicated an inability of the nervous system to block responsivity to excess stimulation. This may have been reflected by these infants' poor ability to regulate state and to signal the examiner that the interaction was inappropriate. It is possible that infants who are hyperalert, irritable, and active or who remain asleep or close their eyes when stimulated for attention are better off because they can communicate that the stimulation is too stressful.

Follow-Up

In the physiology study, on the Bayley Scales at the nine-month follow-up, the term and preterm groups did not differ on the MDI, but the term infants scored higher on the Psychomotor Development Index (PDI). Significant correlations were found between the spectral analysis measures of the heart rate and Bayley MDI and PDI scores, but only during the processing condition. More rhythmic activity in heart rate during newborn attention was related to mental and motor performance at nine months of age.

The fact that the correlations were significant only during attentional processing supports the idea that some behavioral measures may be thought of as a form of stress testing. From an engineering point of view, the best way to learn about a system is to provide a stress and observe the results. It is interesting to speculate that the elicitation of attentional responses in newborn infants, especially preterm infants, may push the infants' limits and engage higher levels of nervous system involvement. By assessing dynamic relationships between the nervous system and behavior, we may provide a more sensitive indicator of the neurophysiological status of the infant.

DISCUSSION

Arthur Parmelee: Barry, as you know, Marian Sigman has written several articles on the visual attention measure with preterms at term and later outcome. She found that preterms looked at the stimulus twice as long as full-term infants, and there was a negative correlation between duration of looking and later outcome. That parallels what you are saying. Whether they are unable to regulate and turn away from the target or whether it's slower information processing is still an issue.

Barry Lester: This is similar to Sigman's findings, although we do not know the quality of the alertness she observed. Initially, I thought she was reporting the kind of hyperalertness that we thought was operating in our low Bayley infants.

Joy Goldberger: It is very reminiscent of the hypervigilance that you expect to see in an infant failing to thrive or an infant who has been in the hospital at an early age, even for a very brief period of time. They become hypervigilant, but with very low affect along with it.

Barry Lester: Can you describe what you mean by hypervigilance?

Joy Goldberger: Very aware of all the movement in the room, focusing quickly on what's happening in the environment. In some ways it looks good; the babies hear a sound and they find it, they orient to it. They're active in that sense, but at the same time it looks like fear, if you were to ascribe a feeling to it. It's a very fearful kind of look.

Barry Lester: When we talked about hyperalertness, we used to talk about the panicky look. But that's not the quality of alertness that we were looking at in these low Bayley babies. Here it was calm, dull, distant, not exaggerated, and not panicky. If anything the affect was absent or flat, with lack of facial participation.

Robert Isaacson: In infant rats and some other animals, any movement produces a heart rate acceleration, even just a slight turn. How much of the heart rate change you found might have been contributed by even relatively small movements?

Barry Lester: With respect to the human, that controversy has been going on for years, as represented by debates between the Laceys and Obrust. While movement certainly can create artifact and acceleration, I think most people now agree that there is a clear information-processing and attention component. In our data, movement artifact would produce the opposite of our findings, because we started with babies quiet, alert, and not moving and presented them with a stimulus. If turning the head produces an increase in heart rate, then they should have shown increases in heart rate from the baseline to the orientation conditions, because they were going from less activity to more activity.

Robert Isaacson: Maybe instead of having a rate-dependent alteration, we ought to think of a state-dependent alteration. If this preterm infant were in an endocrine-activated state, let us say, and you apply a stimulus, you might get a decrease even though the heart rate baseline was the same.

Nico Spinelli: What Bob is referring to is what the psychometricians call systems theory. You have states, you have transition rules that take you from one state to the other, you have input states, and you have output states. State A might have three rules that let you move out of it, and State B might have four rules. Everything is neatly specified. You can do that with machines, and sometimes you can also do it with people. If a person is in shock and you do some things that normally are okay, you'll do him harm. You have different transition rules for each state.

Arthur Parmelee: We've been talking about systems all along—the system in the baby and the system with the environment and the interaction with the environment.

Nico Spinelli: Precisely. Now, psychometricians normally start their papers with a review of systems theory. And somehow even though people around here talk a lot about states, nobody has really defined it. But from that side of the table we keep hearing, "Well, I get different reactions when my babies are in different states. How do I know what to do?" And one concept that is clear in systems theory is that of the transitional rules. I assume this is what your research is trying to get to.

Arthur Parmelee: The system isn't just in the baby, it's the environment of the baby.

Nico Spinelli: Well, that's the whole point of systems theory. Sometimes it's too inclusive; it includes everything.

Arthur Parmelee: We're trying to specify it. That's what we're trying to do.

INFANT STIMULATION: ISSUES OF THEORY AND RESEARCH

Anneliese F. Korner, Ph.D.

If some infant stimulation is beneficial, is more better? If infant stimulation accelerates maturation, does a faster rate of developing certain functions lead to a higher level of functioning in the long run? How should one choose the sensory modalities for infant stimulation? How do individual differences in dealing with stimulation relate to later coping and defense mechanisms and other characteristics of temperament?

These and other questions are explored as this paper addresses the topic of infant stimulation from two different directions: the developmental relevance of stimulation for infants in general and the differences in responsiveness to stimulation on the part of individual infants.

Stimulation and Development

There is currently a lively controversy regarding the benefits and potential hazards of providing stimulation to preterm infants. Until the early 1960s, preterm infants were considered too fragile to tolerate any stimulation, and minimal handling was prescribed in the care of these infants. As time went on, behavioral scientists became very much concerned that preterm infants raised in "isolettes" may be sensorially deprived. Intervention studies were instituted involving a variety of tactile, vestibular-proprioceptive, auditory, visual, and social stimulation, singly or in combination. In the late 1970s, however, we began to learn that instead of being sensorially deprived, preterm infants were bombarded by sensory stimuli, both from the technological environment in which they were raised and from the intensive medical care they were receiving to keep them alive. As a result of these new findings, minimal handling protocols have again become prevalent. Have we come full circle? Perhaps we have, but not quite.

We have learned that not all preterm infants are too fragile to tolerate any stimulation and that responses reflecting physiological or behavioral disorganization result mostly from the aversive, stressful, or noxious stimulation that frequently attends intensive care. We have also learned that preterm infants derive a great variety of benefits from different types of stimulation. The question now is not *whether* stimulation for preterm infants is indicated, but for whom, what kind, how much, at what intervals, at what conceptional age, and for what purpose.

One theoretical controversy stems from differences in the perception of what preterm infants need. On the one hand, preterm infants have frequently been viewed as being deprived of the many forms of stimulation that are prevalent in the natural home environment; on the other hand, they have been seen as deprived of the many different forms of stimulation that are prevalent in utero. Depending on the conceptional age of the infant, a good argument could be made both for and against each of these views. The very young preterm infant may be deprived of the containment and the vestibular-proprioceptive stimulation so prevalent in utero. This does not mean that in providing compensatory stimulation one should try to simulate the intrauterine environment, even if that were possible. Older preterm infants may be deprived of the auditory, visual, and social stimulation of the home environment, but infants born prematurely function differently from full-term infants even when they are of the same conceptional age. We know from studies (for example, Brown & Bakeman, 1979; Field, 1979) that in interactions with their caregivers, infants born prematurely easily become disorganized unless they are handled differently from full-term infants.

If not all preterm infants are too fragile to tolerate stimulation, two very important questions need to be addressed: (1) What purposes might stimulation serve in the development of preterm infants? and (2) Should the choice of the form of stimulation be influenced by the infant's conceptional age? To answer the second question first, it seems indeed important to consider the infant's conceptional age in choosing the modality of stimulation to be given. Studies of both animal and human prenatal development show that the sensory systems appear to mature in an orderly progression, beginning with cutaneous responsitivity in the oral or snout region and progressing to vestibular, auditory, and visual responsivity (Gottlieb, 1971b). Sensory systems begin to function before their structures have completely matured, and there is a reciprocal influence between structure and function (Gottlieb, 1976).

Presumably conditions in utero provide the stimulation necessary for optimizing the outcome of pregnancy. Premature birth must then represent a major and abrupt disruption of this process. It therefore seems to make sense that in designing intervention studies with preterm infants, one should consider which sensory functions were likely disrupted in their development by the premature birth. This will vary, of course, depending on the conceptional age of the infant. To be most effective, stimulation must be maturationally relevant.

From this perspective, one can infer the answer to my question about the purposes that stimulation might serve in the development of preterm infants: in providing stimulation designed to compensate for an experiential deficit by activating maturationally relevant sensory systems, one might assist in the resumption of a process interrupted by premature birth. The goal of sensory stimulation would be to put the infant's development back on track.

Because I hold this view, the aim of my own intervention studies is not to accelerate development but, if possible, to maintain and facilitate it. Thus, it makes sense, to me at least, to use forms of stimulation that activate sensory systems that have matured or are about to mature. In choosing outcome measures, it makes sense to look for gains in the functioning of those systems as well as for the onset of functioning of the sensory systems next in line to mature. With respect to the latter, stimulation of one sensory system can induce the functioning of sensory systems that are about to develop. In several studies (Neal, 1967; Barnard & Bee, 1983; Korner, Schneider, & Forrest, 1983), preterm infants who were provided with vestibular-proprioceptive stimulation began to function better in the auditory and visual spheres than did controls.

The next question is, how does one best implement maturationally relevant sensory stimulation to preterm infants? Such implementation not only requires a knowledge of prenatal development but involves a trial-and-error approach, a little bit of luck, and a great deal of intuitive thinking. Much depends on precisely how such stimulation is imparted. The choices are infinite. Let us take the example of providing vestibular-proprioceptive stimulation, a form of stimulation that is certainly highly relevant for very young preterm infants. Not all movement stimulation should be expected to produce the same results. Yet judging from our first-hand experience with our waterbed studies, this is frequently assumed. Waterbeds can be soft or hard, insulated or not. They can provide containment or not. They can oscillate regularly, irregularly, or intermittently, gently or vigorously, at high or low frequencies, or not at all. Yet it has been widely assumed that all types of waterbeds will have the same effects. In fact, the use of other kinds of beds providing different types of movement stimulation has been justified on the assumption that they would have the same effects as waterbeds.

It is clear from many other examples that effects usually do not generalize and that much depends on precisely how stimulation, even in the same sensory modality, is delivered. For example, in studies of tactile stimulation, very minor changes in kind, quality, quantity, or interval of stimulation can lead to major differences in outcome (see Brown & Martin, 1974; Schanberg, Evoniuk, & Kuhn, 1984).

Outcomes are influenced not only by the kinds of stimulation given and the sensory modalities used but by *how* stimulation is provided. One thing is certain: contrary to prevailing views, more is not better. Much depends on what is to be achieved through stimulation. To soothe an infant, one would provide low, gentle, continuous if not redundant stimulation, no matter what modality is used. To rouse an infant, one would provide more vigorous, faster, and intermittent stimulation.

The last and all-important question is, for whom is infant stimulation indicated? It is probably fair to say that extra stimulation may not be indicated for many infants who are in the process of struggling to achieve some sort of homeostatic equilibrium or who are so weakened by recent severe illness that they cannot deal with even minor challenges. We had an instructive first-hand experience in one of our studies that pointed to this most important problem. In a prior study (Korner et al., 1975) we had found that low-risk preterm infants randomly assigned to waterbeds that gently oscillated in the rhythm of maternal resting respirations had significantly fewer apneas than did controls. In a replication study (Korner et al., 1978), we found confirmation of our previous finding that while the infants were on the oscillating waterbeds, they had significantly less apnea. However, when we looked at the most severe types of apnea as defined by their association with slowing of the heart rate to below eighty beats per minute, we found that one infant's response ran completely counter to that of the group. This infant had many medical problems and we learned a lot from him. We also learned that he was not unique. Highly unstable infants who are being weaned from ventilators or who have major cardiopulmonary or neurological complications and infants treated with theophylline are not likely to respond to waterbeds with apnea reduction (Korner, 1981).

This brings us to the important issue of individual differences in response to stimulation.

Individual Differences

As with the issue of preterm infant stimulation, views on individual differences have undergone several major swings. Until the 1930s psychological thinking was characterized by a very strong belief in individual differences, based largely on the conviction that intelligence was innate and fairly impervious to the influences of early stimulation and experience. The groundbreaking work of Skeels (Skeels et al., 1938) began to sensitize the field to the developmental importance of early stimulation. Skeels placed mentally retarded orphans with institutionalized retarded adults who gave these infants a lot of love, stimulation, and attention. The development of these infants dramatically changed for the better compared with those who remained in the orphanage, and this difference persisted to adulthood (Skeels, 1966). These and other studies gradually but radically changed prevailing child-rearing views, and individual differences in infant responsiveness were all but forgotten. For clinicians, in particular, infant development depended on what mothers did with or to their babies and on the amount and quality of early stimulation to which the infants were exposed.

During this period, only a small group of investigators and theoreticians were concerned with the issue of innate or congenital individual differences. Interestingly, most of these workers were influenced by Freud, who, in spite of all his writings on the effects of early experience, was a strong believer in innate individual characteristics. Psychoanalytic thinking sparked the early infant observations of Escalona (Escalona et al., 1952, 1963) and Brazelton's (1962, 1973) studies of early individuality of neonates. In fact, Brazelton's observations with the Neonatal Behavioral Assessment Scale (1973) have not only alerted the world to the newborn's exquisite responsivity to stimulation but helped to turn around psychoanalytic thinking, particularly about the innate "stimulus barrier" of newborns. They showed that rather than warding off all external stimulation in the service of maintaining homeostasis, as Freud thought, newborns seek external stimulation and ward it off only when for internal reasons it becomes too intense, and that there are vast individual differences in both these needs.

My own research of individual differences at birth was also strongly influenced by psychoanalytic theory (Korner, 1964, 1971). My interest originated with clinical work with young children and their families, which led me to want to investigate the origins of the defense mechanisms. Characteristic ways of dealing with or warding off stimulation and of managing excitation seemed to me the central issue in the development of the defense mechanisms and coping strategies. I hypothesized that the infant's response to stimulation may be an early behavioral manifestation of individual differences in CNS functioning and that such differences might well determine how much stimulation individual infants needed and how much they could tolerate.

I therefore attempted for many years to study individual differences in sensory thresholds and the regulatory mechanisms with which normal, full-term newborns can respond to stimulation. Even though our studies reflected highly significant differences in response to stimuli, we found that the reliability of measurements of sensory responsiveness was readily compromised by the smallest fluctuations in the infant's state (Korner, 1972). We therefore turned to assessing motor output rather than sensory thresholds in response to sensory stimulation. In order to study individual differences in activity patterns and characteristic levels of energy output, we developed an electronic neonatal activity monitor. In our studies, we not only found highly significant stability of motor behavior (Korner et al., 1981), but we also found significant relations between the vigor of motions at birth and the later activity and temperament of the same children at four to eight years of age (Korner et al., 1985).

It was not until the late 1970s and early 1980s that individual differences in reaction patterns became widely accepted as an important subject to study in their own right. We appear now to be in the middle of another historical swing, in which we tend to devalue earlier approaches to the study of development involving the search for main effects.

Implications for Research

In providing infant stimulation, we need to make a clear distinction between clinical intervention and efficacy research. In clinical intervention, the soundest way to proceed is to try to tailor stimulation to what we perceive to be the individual needs and characteristics of each infant. In this context, one is free to change one's approach if the infant does not respond favorably, and this is exactly how it should be. But this approach has an important drawback. With each infant being exposed to an individualized treatment approach, it is often difficult to see clearly which factors in the infant or in the treatment are responsible for some infants' failing to respond.

The research question posed in clinical intervention is: "Given a stimulation protocol tailored to the individual needs of different infants, how many of them respond favorably?" The question posed in efficacy research is quite different: "Does a particular form of stimulation benefit infants?" Obviously, both research approaches have their own validity and assets. We really need more balance and perspective in our thinking and should not abandon what some consider to be old approaches for "newly discovered" ones that usually are not all that new. Let us not forget that controlled experimental studies that seek to test the main effects produced by uniform research protocols have distinct advantages. By using a randomized design that precludes bias of selection, we can gain a great deal of systematic knowledge about whether or not a given form of stimulation works and about the individual characteristics that cause some infants to fail to respond. Only with a standard treatment protocol as provided in controlled, randomized experimental studies will the factors inherent in the infants who failed to respond stand out clearly.

DISCUSSION

Peter Gorski: How long should the intervention persist to get lasting results? That is a major practical concern.

Anneliese Korner: I am not nearly as concerned about lasting effects as I am about what this intervention alleviates right then and there. Does it help the soundness of sleep? Does it alleviate apnea? Whom does it help and whom doesn't it? All one needs to do is to read the literature to see how few lasting effects there are as a result of any intervention. If there are beneficial long-term effects, that is great. But if there are not, I am not surprised. We know there are much more powerful experiences than the exposure to a waterbed for ten or twenty days. The familial and the socioeconomic influences on development are so powerful that few things we do persist. I think we are very hung up on the whole issue of whether intervention will affect development from here on in.

Barry Lester: Certainly clinicians and funding agencies are.

Anneliese Korner: But we shouldn't fall in with a funding agency on that. It's not that I think we shouldn't be interested in long-term effects. It's just that we should know by now that we can't count on them. I think that there is an incredible devaluation of current beneficial effects. People think nothing is any good unless there are permanent changes. It's like saying you shouldn't feed people because this may not increase their eventual IQs. If you benefit the child, then you can build upon that benefit.

Craig Ramey: There seems to be a contradiction in the attempt on the one hand to demonstrate plasticity on the behavioral or neurological level, and on the other hand, to ask that an intervention produce a permanent effect, especially when we define "permanent" in such a strange way. Usually when we look for enduring effects, we end up measuring quite different behaviors from what we attempted to change with our interventions. So we're not asking whether the thing that we have changed remains changed—do you continue to reduce apnea edisodes? Instead the question gets enlarged, and we ask for some generalized improvement. And if development were so plastic that we were able to produce a permanent change by a relatively small, early intervention, then we would also seem to imply that early insults that have any significance would also be likely to have negative effects. I'm just underscoring your point that the search for permanent effects seems to be uninformed by theory. I know of no theory in psychology that predicts permanence of change. I think if you make that point, it will turn out to be a profound one.

Tiffany Field: From your perspective, Anneliese, with the dramatic effects you've shown, why do you suppose that waterbeds haven't been adopted widely?

Anneliese Korner: Actually they have been adopted in many places.

Tiffany Field: I know of at least one neonatologist who won't have them on his unit. Even though he knows your data, he's not convinced. I'm just wondering what kind of resistance we're up against with the neonatologists.

Kathryn Barnard: I have a post-doctoral student, Dr. Kris Kaufman-Swanson, who is doing qualitative analysis on some of the beliefs of parents, neonatologists, and nurses who work with me in ICU. In her interviews what is coming across very strongly is the philosophy to do no harm and avoid bad outcomes. We don't even talk about good outcomes. The preoccupation is with avoiding bad outcomes. In relationship to Tiffany's question about why more people aren't using the waterbeds, I think that the infants are so fragile that you do develop a sense of protectiveness in wanting to avoid any bad outcomes. One of the reasons neonatologists and nurses are hesitant is that we expect them to take the findings from one study and apply the techniques or the stimulation program in a clinical way, which then is not studied. We need many more replications of the studies in early interventions than are now happening.

Anneliese Korner: I appreciate that neonatologists don't want to incorporate something into their care that they feel is not proven. I'm much more concerned about the opposite: that they assume that something has been proved and they start using it. When we developed the waterbeds, we did the first study purely as a safety study, to see whether it was safe to put babies on waterbeds for days at a time. We were reassured that nothing was changed except that the infants on the waterbeds experienced apnea reduction. We have since done studies to see what these devices do—what they help and their potential hazards. But to our chagrin, when we published the first paper people thought that the benefits of the waterbed were established definitively.

A very interesting example of how things get incorporated uncritically simply because they make a lot of sense is the result of a sheepskin study that was done in Great Britain on six babies. One can hardly go into any nursery where babies are not on sheepskins. Sometimes, of course, they are not sheepskin but are made of nylon. No one knows whether these results generalize, but people adopt things that are simple to incorporate, that make intuitive sense.

TARGETING INFANT STIMULATION EFFORTS: THEORETICAL CHALLENGES FOR RESEARCH AND INTERVENTION

Frances Degen Horowitz, Ph.D.

Despite the growth of our knowledge about the human infant and the advances in care, our understanding of the factors actually responsible for the developmental course and outcome of individual infants still places heavy reliance on the gross, summary variables that Sameroff and Chandler (1975) identified in the early 1970s: maternal education and socioeconomic status. Siegel's impressive longitudinal study of the preterm infant (Siegel, 1982a, 1982b, 1985; Siegel et al., 1982) puts the major risk indicators in the environmental factors of maternal education and socioeconomic status and in the perinatal events of apnea and asphyxia. While such a risk index allows us to make better predictions, it puts us no nearer to an understanding of the processes responsible for outcome.

With respect to the preterm infant, after more than fifteen years of research on early stimulation there are still many questions that remain and some increasing doubts about the advisability of blanket early stimulation interventions in the NICU. Many participating in this Round Table are asking whether early stimulation is always desirable, whether it may not be more prudent to ask *when*, *what kind*, and *for what goal*—although there are no more satisfactory or certain answers to these more limited approaches.

This paper places the concerns about early stimulation in a broader developmental context, drawing on an analysis that is both selective and eclectic.

Theoretical Considerations

The major theories that have guided much of our thinking in behavioral development can be found in Gesell, Freud, behaviorism, and Piaget and the cognitivists. The basic concepts that inform much of the empirical research can be traced to one or another of these general theoretical orientations. And each can be said to touch upon elements that, if selectively sampled and combined, may provide a clearer picture to guide our research into the processes that account for developmental outcome.

When these major theories were originally formulated, mostly in the 1920s and 1930s, much less was known about infant behavior and development, the survival rate of premature infants was significantly lower, and "high-risk" and "at-risk" were not in the lexicon. Yet Gesell's work was strongly oriented to infant development. He maintained a staunch neuromaturational point of view, citing the strong influence of heredity and the stability of individual differences. He gave little weight to the effect of specific environmental interventions or the efficacy of special learning opportunities.

The behaviorists were interested in infants as a proving ground for the laws of conditioning. The notion was that if you could demonstrate that infants could learn, then the proposition that behavioral development was largely a function of learned associations would be viable.

Piaget was already at work describing the sensorimotor period of development, but his work had little impact on Gesell or the behaviorists and was generally ignored by Americans. Freud's influence was extensive, especially in relation to early psychosexual development, but his ideas were not the subject of extensive empirical test except when translated by behavioristically oriented psychologists examining social learning. Freud's emphasis upon socioemotional development and the importance of early infant experience for shaping later development was compatible with behavioristic analysis of learned associations and relationships.

Gesell's influence waned after the 1940s, and the behavioristic point of view gained dominance. Infants were seen as learning organisms, and Neal Miller (1959) observed that the human organism came into the world especially prepared to learn. This observation was prescient in that it was made at a time when little was known about the sensory and stimulus-processing capabilities of the newborn and young infant. The stimulus-response analysis, especially that advanced by Skinner and the operant psychologists, has produced the strongest body of behavioral laws we currently have, the most applicable to the treatment of specific behavioral problems and the most amenable to empirical test. It does not, however, represent the only valid scientific track.

In fact, behavioristic analysis has in general been less developmentally oriented than other points of view and also less tied to the structural characteristics of organisms. One of the attractions of the cognitivist and systems theory perspectives is that they do attempt to encompass the species-specific structural complexities that contribute to the development course of an organism. These perspectives are difficult to investigate empirically, but they are a rich source of hypotheses for deriving studies of interactional relationships and their effect on behavioral development.

It is possible and profitable to develop a point of view encompassing the strengths of both the behaviorist analysis and the cognitive/evolutionary orientation. This ecumenical approach is not new, but a fully developmental analysis that melds these different perspectives has been attempted only recently (Horowitz, in press).

A Structural/Behavioral Analysis

Figure 6 is an attempt to describe the sources and elements that must be built into any model of behavioral development. At the center, C represents conception. It is surrounded by a somewhat oval-shaped line with the intersect of B, for birth. Behavioral and structural development is posited as the result of the interplay between the information coded in the genes and environmental events, even during the period between conception and birth. The forces that impact on development are represented by dotted and solid lines showing relationships that have three aspects: (1) a rough pattern of sequences and stages, the gross topography of which fixes human behavior patterns; (2) the periodic organization and reorganization of these patterns under conditions of relevant environmental stimulation; and (3) the various sources and levels of that stimulation. These forces that influence development include the basic physical principles that govern the environment; culture,

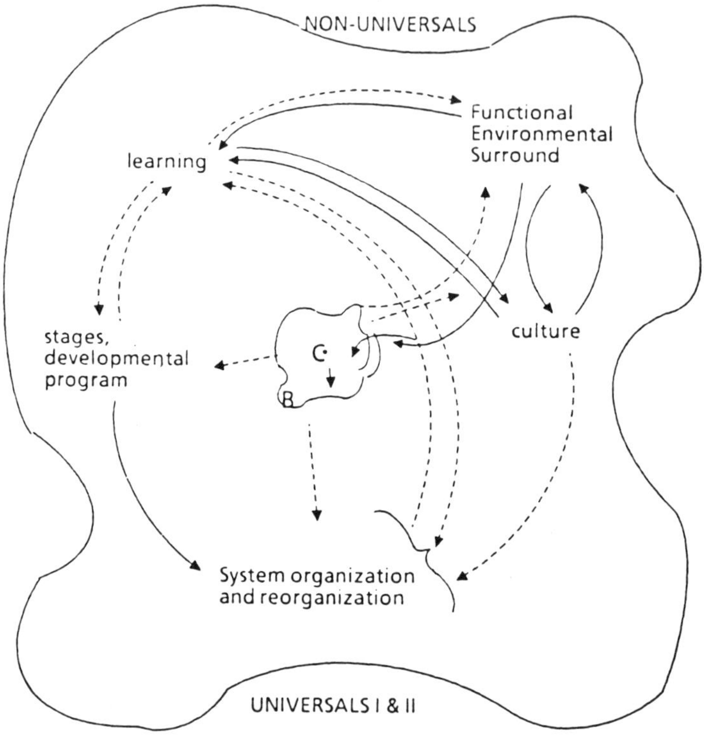

Figure 6. A model of behavioral development

defined as the overriding organization patterns of the environment that emphasize some aspects of the environment over others; patterns of saliencies, which are at once subtle and pervasive in the experience of an individual developing in that culture; and organized patterns of stimulation that are contingent upon behaviors defined as opportunities for learning.

The behavioral repertoire developed as a result of these interacting components involves three distinct classes of behaviors: Universals I, Universals II, and Non-universals. Universal I behaviors are those that might be said to be "hard-wired," extremely probable behaviors that develop over a short period of time. Indeed, these behaviors may have nearly completed their developmental course by birth or shortly thereafter. Examples of Universal I behaviors are found in the sensory perceptual domains. Defects in these behaviors will largely be traced to specific neurological dysfunction and are not easily corrected by environmental stimulation. While these behaviors do not require much by way of environmental stimulation for development, they do require a basic functional environment for their maintenance and for their integration into other types of behaviors.

Universal II behaviors are those highly probable behaviors that develop over a longer period of time. They require not only a functional ambient environment but specific environmental stimulus feedback to shape the behavior, which is species- specific. The level of development attained and the integration of the behaviors with other types of behaviors depend upon specific learning opportunities and culturally determined emphases. The Piagetian sensorimotor intelligence behaviors are of this kind. Their acquisition is highly probable in the normal human organism in the normal environment. The processes that account for their development involve a combination of organismically determined topographies and sequences, perhaps state and system organizations inherent to the species, and stimulus-response packages of contingent feedback that contribute to the shape of the behaviors.

Universal II behaviors include many of the behaviors cited to support the case for a programmed unfolding of behavioral development that is relatively invariant from child to child. In this analysis the general topography and sequence of those behaviors is invariant, but not the level of achievement, the rate of acquisition, the quality of the behavior, and its eventual integration with Non-universal behaviors.

Non-universal behaviors are all those behaviors that are the result of specific learning opportunities and cultural emphases. They probably account, ultimately, for the largest portion of the human behavioral repertoire and are theoretically unlimited.

The Behavioral Organization of the Infant

The structural/behavior analysis that has been described here can contribute to an understanding of infant behavior and development and to the issues of early stimulation for the preterm infant. Between conception and birth, the development of the gross behavioral topographies and the developmental trajectories of those behaviors are highly specified. Given a normal genetic endowment, a normal prenatal environment, and a normally functioning host, the probability is high that the normal behavioral repertoire of the human newborn will in fact develop.

The organization of the behavioral repertoire here classified as Universal II is also somewhat determined. A critical variable affecting the organization of the behavior and the ultimate smoothness of its patterning and functioning involves state. While we do not have an analysis of state in the human organism beyond the period of infancy, it has become increasingly clear that state and state organization may be the overriding behavioral component during infancy, especially during the neonatal period and early infancy.

State regulation in neonates has been reported to predict developmental outcome (Tynan, 1986; Thoman, Miano, & Freese, 1977; Thoman et al., 1979, Thoman & Becker, 1979; Colombo, 1986). The role of state and state organization and state stability may be complex in relation to development. One possibility is that state and state organization may influence the acquisition of Universal II behaviors, affecting the ease with which they develop, the rate of development, and their early elaboration in relation to Non-universal behaviors. State may influence the general organization of early behavior in the normal healthy term infant during the neonatal period, and an assessment of state such as the Brazelton Neonatal Behavioral Assessment Scale (NBAS) provides may be a part of the predictive equation accounting for developmental outcome. With the preterm infant, state may be an even more significant variable. The younger and sicker the preterm infant, the more central a variable it may be.

Behavioral variability, which may very well be related to state, has been shown to be a critical variable in mother-infant interaction. Linn and Horowitz (1983) reported that infants with greater behavioral variability on the NBAS were more likely to be involved in an interaction with a responsive mother. Behavioral variability may be a positive indicator of relatively better state control, or it may elicit more state-organizing behaviors on the part of the caregiver. The consistent finding of socioeconomic status and maternal education as predictors of developmental outcome may reflect the fact that higher-SES caregivers and those with more education have a broader behavioral repertoire for fostering good state organization in infants. In other words, the early role of the mother or caregiver in interacting with the infant may not be so much in providing specific kinds of stimulation but in being able to draw on behaviors that help the infant organize and modulate behavioral state. This perspective has some important implications for early stimulation of high-risk infants.

Early Stimulation and the High-Risk Infant

Almost all preterm infants born in the United States now receive some sort of special care in a special nursery. This environment and the infant's interactions with it have come under increased scrutiny in the last several years. Almost all the interest has focused upon the effects of various types of early stimulation—waterbeds, handling, visual and auditory stimuli.

Where the interventions have been shown to be beneficial, it is likely that they had their effects by helping the infant to organize state and thus fostering the maturation of the central nervous system (CNS). This would suggest that the question we ought to ask is, what type of stimulation, and with what timing, is successful in helping the infant with state organization? At certain points the functional state organization may be to increase the stability of state; closer to term and with greater CNS maturity, the most functional organization of state may be to foster smooth state-to-state transitions and to enable the infant to handle state variability.

State stability may promote the development of the general topography of Universal II behaviors. The more mature handling of state variability and state transition may permit higher levels of achievement of these behaviors and increase the acquisition of the early non-universal behaviors.

The overriding implication of this analysis is that early stimulation of high-risk infants needs to be analyzed in terms of fostering state organization (both stability and variability) and in terms of the level of CNS maturation and the relative needs for state stability and variability at different points in development. Thus, the specific content of the stimulation may be less important, especially in the earliest months of life, than whether or not the stimulation facilitates state organization.

It is probably not an accident that many of the normal maternal ministering behaviors in early infancy involve facilitation of state modulation. The aversive nature of infant cries may have an evolutionarily adaptive function in eliciting the kind of caregiving behaviors that stimulate state organization. As we have noted, more highly educated mothers may have a greater set of skills from which to draw in order to do this, and this factor may be the initial source of the relationship between maternal education and developmental outcome. In much of the research now going on in mother-infant interaction, especially where videotapes are available, it would be useful to focus on the degree and extent of the mother's skills in modulating infant organization and transitions. If this turns out to be fruitful, it will give us a knowledge base that will permit us to target early stimulation interventions. Additionally, the specific inability of mothers and other caretakers to modulate state behavior and promote state organization in young infants may be a strong predictor of child abuse behaviors.

It is quite possible that state-organization stimulation is most relevant to the development of Universal II behaviors and that a more content-oriented stimulation program is most relevant to the development of Non-universal behaviors. This would mean that early stimulation programs need to be shaped in terms of targeted behaviors. Early stimulation for infants at risk socioeconomically might properly be designed with regard to specific content experiences—visual, auditory, kinesthetic, and vestibular. The target would be to expand and elaborate the child's knowledge base of the world in order to build upon the Universal II behavior repertoire. The infant more physically at risk might well benefit from an early stimulation program that is targeted on fostering state modulation, especially in the earliest days and months, and that later shades over to a more content-oriented intervention. This perspective calls for a somewhat different research agenda on early stimulation and high-risk infants than we have been pursuing.

DISCUSSION

Craig Ramey: I was delighted to hear in your comments the recognition that different kinds of children need different forms of intervention. That has not been universally recognized. You also implied that intervention has different purposes. For example, a child from a very disadvantaged and impoverished background, may need a general kind of enrichment, to provide supports across the developmental terrain, whereas a child who has a very specific developmental deficit may need a program tailored to that particular deficit. But as we look across the intervention literature over the past quarter of a century, the only measure that intervention programs have taken in common is a local measure of intellectual function. And that measure has been taken at different points in development depending on when the intervention was instituted and when it was stopped. As everyone here is aware, those tests at different points in development tap fundamentally different processes. We should not delude ourselves into thinking that that measurement at age three is necessarily tapping the same process that we tap at age three months or at age five years.

All of which leads me to ask this question: Since we have such a dilemma in trying to relate various levels of intervention to a common outcome that is itself very complex, can you provide some guidance as to the kind of criteria one might use to guide the selection of developmental outcome measures?

Frances Horowitz: I don't think I can answer that just off the top of my head. What you're saying is absolutely right. But I don't have a quick answer to it.

Craig Ramey: I don't have a quick answer, either—or a long one. It seems to me that the problem is the lack of a specific model that traces the intended effect, or traces a particular intervention through a series of mechanisms to some outcome. I think we could do ourselves a great deal of good by putting as much effort into prespecifying the intended course of our intervention as in collecting the broadest array of data that we can.

Nico Spinelli: Are you saying that there is no way to evaluate success?

Frances Horowitz: There are some very limited ways to evaluate success. We put a great deal of store in various intellectual measures, but as far as styles or social and emotional development are concerned, except in the psychiatric literature, there is a paucity of material in our measurement bank.

I think of developmental outcome as the result of an equation, and one of our problems is that we don't know all the variables that go into the equation, much less how to weight them. Moreover, over the course of development,the nature of that equation may change. We need to trace the degree to which process is the same over periods of development and the junctures at which process may change. In some domains you're going to get stronger continuities than in other domains. Some environmental interventions may be much more effective if they are delayed, because they are more relevant to the equation that will be functioning at a later time.

Craig Ramey: As a first step, it would do us well to examine the specific behaviors that a measure is tapping. If we're giving a Stanford-Binet at age five as one of our major outcome measures, a content analysis of what the Stanford-Binet taps as psychological processes at age five might help us to understand what we have done to change this outcome. Because if we do the same content analysis on the Bayley Scale at 24 months, we will find we are dealing with fundamentally different behaviors. And we can stop short of doing a conceptual analysis. We could simply analyze what behaviors we are asking the child to exhibit in order to be judged competent. Frequently we don't do even that step.

Frances Horowitz: I'd like to come back to a comment that Anneliese made about being concerned with contemporaneous effects. There may be a number of environmental factors that operate only for contemporaneous effects that are very important to the organism but that we do not expect to have any permanent or long-term outcome. There may be other environmental aspects that are very important for the long-term effects. For example, most of us tend to think of an early enriched language environment as important to the subsequent level of language competence. I think we need to sort out what we do with children and what environmental components there are in terms of our expectations, and at the present we do not have a good theoretical guideline for that.

Barry Lester: Language is a good example, because presumably your intervention is going to intervene in a similar function, where you want to affect the outcome of that same function or process. I think that's the most simple-minded answer to your question, Craig. If you want to do intervention on a function, then your developmental outcome should measure the same function.

Craig Ramey: We must be careful, however. I think language is a wonderful metaphor, because it's one of the Universals. It's also one of the Non-universals—it shares characteristics across your classification system. If we do an intervention program, we should be very careful that we haven't intervened at, say, the semantic level during the period of language acquisition and then measured the success of the intervention in terms of a pragmatic level of assessment done three years later. We're asking for an extraordinary generalization. We're not testing on items that are similar to what was taught; we're generalizing even further than that, to a different realm in language functioning. Of all the problems in psychology that people are now working on, I think generalization is the toughest one. Frequently we measure the effects of interventions by going to horrendous levels of generalization. So your analogy to language is apt, and it also contains within it the seeds of complexity of the problem.

Nico Spinelli: For those of us who'd like to be simple-minded and come up with simply measured numbers, could it be said, for example, that a mother or a therapist faced with a premature baby who is exhibiting high cardiac rate variance has the goal to reduce that variance? There's a measure of success. I'd like to have a clear-cut measure of success. Would that be one?

Peter Vietze: We don't know if reduced heart rate variance means anything at that age.

Nico Spinelli: Right. So there are many things that one could measure, but the fact is that on any one dimension one is not clear what those measures mean.

Peter Vietze: I think the reason Fran answered you as she did is that in developmental psychology we've been talking about process measures, and we haven't really been developing them. There are increasingly good cognitive processing measures for school-age children and now even for adolescents, but the problem is that we don't know how they relate to other things. We don't know how they relate to smartness.

Edward Tronick: It's not the problem of finding measures; there are a lot of things to measure. The question, especially when we want to do some intervention, is to evaluate whether the outcome is indeed positive. We can reduce bradycardia; the question then becomes, is that what we want to be doing? To take the radical example of the infants in Peru, which is a qualitatively different kind of example, one can say that their goal is acclimatization, getting the babies' thermal regulatory mechanisms in place. And they do it in a particular kind of way. That's quite positive, but it also probably has some negative effects. We could then evaluate that, or ask if it is really positive.

Frances Horowitz: I want to say something about our outcome measures, because I see that you thought I was evading the question. I'm reminded of an experience that was very sobering to me, when we were involved in the 1960s in the national evaluation of the effect of Head Start. I remember one meeting in Washington in which the only outcome measure being proposed was IQ. A number of us argued against the IQ for lots of reasons. Finally the person in charge said, "Look, this is the only thing that Congress will understand, and if you don't use IQ, you're going to destroy the program." Well, it turned out, as a result of this massive evaluation, that there was an IQ difference that was highly significant, because you had thousands of children; the difference was about five IQ points. It was a totally nonfunctional outcome, as far as we know. And yet it's turned out that a number of the more highly controlled, high quality, intervention programs had other very interesting long-term outcomes that had absolutely nothing to do with IQ but with functional behavior in society.

IQ is there because we've got it and everyone understands what it is, but I hope that in fifty years we won't be using IQ any more, that we'll understand enough about intellectual processing and intellectual function that we'll have other, different measures. I wasn't just being evasive. I don't accept what I think of as our very simple-minded dependence upon the one outcome measure that people understand, and I think it has basically deterred us from identifying outcome measures that are much, much more meaningful in terms of human behavior.

PART III
INTERVENTION

INFANTS ON ACUTE CARE HOSPITAL UNITS: ISSUES IN STIMULATION AND INTERVENTION

Joy Goldberger, M.S.

Much attention has been focused on stimulation needs of preterm infants and on intervention programs for high-risk and handicapped infants. Yet informal estimates suggest that 50 percent of pediatric hospital beds are filled by children under two years of age, many of whom are not in neonatal intensive care units. A large percentage are admitted to pediatric units that may or may not provide environments, facilities, services, and caregivers geared toward the unique needs of infants and their families (Wagner & McCue, 1987).

Many of these infants and toddlers have complex medical needs and require extended hospital care. Many experience repeated hospital admissions. Little attention is directed at defining and providing for the emotional and developmental needs of infants in hospitals. Yet Douglas (1975), in his landmark study of the behavioral and learning sequelae to hospitalization, considered children between seven months and three years to be the most likely to suffer temporary and long-term disturbances that often persist into adolescence. Infants less than six months of age hospitalized longer than one week were found to have signficantly greater instability in job patterns in adolescence. Infants from seven months to one year of age hospitalized for longer than one week were found to have a greater rate of reading problems and delinquency than the general population, and those from one to two years at hospitalization exhibited more "troublesome behavior" in school. Other investigators (Quinton & Rutter, 1976; Meijer, 1985) have reported similar findings.

This paper reviews the many ways in which the hospital environment differs from the home environment of the infant. It then discusses the implications of these differences for the hospital care of infants and in particular for stimulation programs designed for hospitalized infants.

The Home and Hospital Environments of the Infant

Hospitalization may be a profoundly disruptive experience, whether it is predicted or unpredicted, brief or extended, immediately following birth or after patterns of nurturing and attachment have been established. Typically it affects a number of patterns of stimulation and interaction.

Number of caregivers. During the immediate neonatal period, in the "normal" home environment, caregivers include mother and father, often grandparents, aunts, and uncles, and perhaps a babysitter or a sibling or two. Later, the infant experiences visits with others in addition to immediate family and routine childcare providers.

This situation contrasts greatly with the large numbers of people in hospitals who provide care in a variety of styles of interactions. One estimate is that the typical pediatric admission may meet 54 caregivers within the first 24 hours of hospitalization. Grant (1983) observed an average of 327 separate entrances by 106 different people to a six-bed pediatric patient room during a 12-hour period. Smith (1976), observing 18-month-old to five-year-old patients, found that interactions between staff and patients lasted an average of less than 1.5 minutes. Each of these caregivers delivers care with an inevitable individuality of style.

Family stress and vulnerability may compromise the parents' ability to be emotionally responsive or even physically available as caregivers in the hospital. The parents may be experiencing grief, fear, self-doubt, guilt, anger, and conflict over the child's illness. The care of other children at home remains a responsibility. Grandparents may be supportive or may offer opinions that increase conflict. For parents with little education or low socioeconomic resources, the hospital world may seem foreign and hostile.

Encouragement of rhythmicity. At home, rhythmic patterns of day and night are encouraged. Sequences of caregiving are established, such as the timing of baths and of playtime. The cycle of comfort→discomfort→crying→parent intervention that reestablishes comfort is repeated, usually with increasing ease. Parents enjoy and encourage the maintenance of states of awake/alert and sleep.

In hospitals, rhythms and patterns in caregiving are frequently interrupted for medical care. Feeding patterns may be significantly altered. The rhythmic pattern of hunger→crying→feeding and social stimulation→comfort may be absent. Sleep may be the most frequently disrupted pattern. Beardslee (1976) observed children two to five years of age and found problems of wakefulness to be greatly increased when the child's room is close to service areas or when the child has had two or more stressful experiences that day. Hagemann (1981b) compared internal disruptions (physiological needs or discomfort) with external disruptions such as environmental stimuli and caregiving functions and found that nearly two-thirds of the disruptions were externally induced. Moreover, they occurred with such frequency that very few children were observed to sleep without interruption through more than half an expected sleep period.

Responses to infant's cues. In the home environment, the infant's cues are ideally followed by near-immediate responses. Cries bring about feeding, changing, holding, and social and sensory stimulation that are satisfying to the infant. As the infant teaches the parents about what feels right and good to him, the parents in turn are encouraging interaction involving the infant's increasing developmental skills. The fabric of the infant's and the parents' lives become more richly woven, with both interaction and time alone to pursue goals.

In hospitals, the infant's crying may not be responded to evenly by busy staff or by the stressed, fearful family. Parents may be preoccupied with negotiating the hospital system. If the hospital stay is long, or if there are other young children at home, they may be decreasingly available physically or emotionally.

Coordinated multisensory events. Most caregiving at home involves a wealth of coordinated sensory experiences that are repeated with similar organization. For example, feeding simultaneously includes seeing the caregiver and food source, hearing the caregiver's voice, smelling the scent of the caregiver's body, tasting the formula or breast milk, as well as the physical sensations of touch, kinesthetic changes of position, and hunger pains alleviated. Caregivers' and others' voices enable the infant to track them visually.

During hospitalization, sensory events are all too frequently fragmentized. For example, nasogastric feeding breaks the typically coordinated event of eating into discrete parts, of which several—sucking and tasting, being held—are missing. Many environmental sounds are out of the infant's visual field, inhibiting the infant's ability to coordinate sounds with source or movement. Overwhelming auditory input may be "tuned out." Restraints may be used that inhibit instinctual hand movements and self-comforting and pleasurable motor activity.

Older infants, with more extended periods of alert attention, develop more complex needs. These include:

Predictability. Familiar people and routines take on increasing importance for the infant, both cognitively and emotionally. In the home setting, this includes such examples as "When I wake up, I will see Daddy. Baths come after breakfast. When Mommy holds me just this way, I will eat. I sleep here."

Routine caregiving in hospitals, by contrast, is diverse in its presentation and may be perceived as unpredictable. Medical interventions are even less predictable in their style and timing. Room assignment and location of bed may change. The cost of increased social adaptability in chronically hospitalized infants may be increased emotional passivity and diminished self-expression (for example, the chronically ill baby who learns to smile while in pain).

Cause and effect. Cause and effect experiences become increasingly interesting as the infant learns some control over the environment. At home, examples of cause and effect are plentiful: "When I cry I am fed. When I say 'baba' I get a bottle. When I cry and kick my feet my sister stops playing with me."

What is within reach of or controlled by a baby in a hospital crib? The infant can rarely pursue an interesting task and practice concentration and perseverance without interruption. Nor are engrossing, increasingly complex opportunities usually available in the hospital. For many sick infants, learning new skills may require more energy than he can spare. Use of hand restraints, physical restraint by caregivers during procedures, restraint resulting from medical equipment, the effects of fear or depression, and lack of experience with available play materials further combine to decrease spontaneous play and exploration.

Variety. At home, there are interesting and novel changes in environment. Excursions to the supermarket, to homes of family and neighbors, and to social gatherings invite practice and modification of skills and behaviors and encourage exploration, learning, and interaction. Novel situations that are stressful are often time-limited and perhaps serve to develop competence in coping behaviors.

Hospital environments, however, offer few changes over time. New experiences are likely to be trips to surgery or medical tests. In settings where the provision and maintenance of toys are not necessarily any one person's responsibility, play materials may be changed infrequently. One or two rooms and a hallway or two may be the child's unvarying environment for days, weeks, or months at a time.

Personal space. For healthy babies, there are few individuals who have intimate contact with the infant's body. When social interaction is wanted, the infant finds a way to initiate interaction that the family reinforces; when the interaction is no longer pleasurable, ideally the baby turns or moves away or otherwise disengages from the interaction, and the parent changes or terminates the activity.

By contrast, the hospitalized baby's body is touched by many people, often uncomfortably. Usually the infant cannot move away from uncomfortable stimulation or social or physical overstimulation. Staff members who want to feel that they have nurtured rather than hurt a sick infant may engage in excessive tickling or coaxing of smiles when an infant does not feel like smiling. Over-passivity is a costly but highly functional adaptation, as is gaze aversion with an artificial-seeming smile to satisfy too numerous social demands.

Age-appropriate play materials and exploration. In the home environment play materials are optimally presented in a manner that encourages emerging skills without creating undue frustration. Ideally, the majority of toys are available for direct manipulation and exploration and are safe for mouthing and handling. They invite multisensory involvement (auditory, visual, gross and fine motor qualities), and they offer increasing cognitive complexity. The mobile infant has frequent opportunities to move about safely and freely and to explore the immediate environment.

In hospitals, even when toys are available, they are frequently not quite in reach or in the infant's line of vision. Toys that are adequately interesting may be too heavy for a weak infant. Over time, toys lose pieces or are broken. Busy staff may not have time for providing and adapting toys, or budgets may not allocate the funds to acquire them.

Stimulation Programs: Pros and Cons

In some hospitals, programs to facilitate and encourage developmental competence are provided by Nursing, Child Life, Occupational Therapy, or visiting teachers through the local school system. Many provide valuable support for infants and their families; others are potentially counterproductive.

Stimulation programs function best when a primary goal is to provide as many comforts of home as possible and to recognize that parents are nearly always the ideal providers of care and stimulation. The environment and policies are welcoming and nurturing to parents as well as to patients. The staff is *enabling* ("Look how she watches you while we're talking!") rather than *instructive* ("You should talk to her when she's awake") and *supportive* ("Look at that special smile he has just for you") rather than *competitive* ("Look how I've taught him to play peek-a-boo"). Private family time without interruptions from staff but with staff close by for support is beneficial, especially when the setting encourages visits by siblings.

In addition to maximizing parents' comfort and sense of competence, well-coordinated stimulation programs ideally provide developmentally appropriate and skill-encouraging play materials. These should aim to help parents perceive areas of health and potential in their infant and should compensate for restraint and immobility, temporary or chronic disability, environmental monotony, and the baby's need and desire to manipulate, explore, and experience success and competence. Simple adaptations in methods of presenting standard play materials and a creative eye toward alternative toys for special-needs children are essential. A variety of materials should be available to patients and their parents 24 hours a day, rather than just when a "stimulation specialist" is in attendance.

An important facet of the quality of the infant or toddler's hospitalization experience is likely to be the skill and caring of a primary nurse in helping to regulate a rhythmic, predictable routine for her patients, with as few caregivers and interruptions as possible. Along with the parents, the primary nurse can be instrumental in insuring that the infant's comfort, medical condition, emotional needs, and state of arousal take precedence over a discrete, intentional intervention for "stimulation."

For all their good intentions, stimulation programs or practitioners frequently employ practices that are not optimal. A few caveats follow:

1. Stimulation programs or intervention protocols that in tone are analogs to medical procedures may be counterproductive. These may include stimulation "done to" a passive "patient"; events that interrupt sleep-wake cycles or postpone a needed rest time; activities that follow a "prescription" rather than building and flowing between infant and caregiver; and "stimulation" that is not naturally interesting and enjoyable to the child.

2. Parents' confidence may be undermined if they interpret the presence of a stimulation specialist to mean that their infant requires a trained specialist for stimulation and that without professional assistance they would not be adequate to care for their child's sensory nurturing and normal development. Similarly, parents' perception of their infant may be negatively affected when deficits rather than capabilities are focused upon.

3. Spending an infant's energy in adult-designed tasks has often seemed to decrease a sick infant's ability to attend to, respond to, and cope with environmental stimulation and has seemed to decrease some babies' ability to organize those skills already mastered.

4. Some designers of stimulation programs combine collected research protocols into programs that may have unknown effects and could be potentially overwhelming or otherwise dangerous to a medically fragile infant.

5. Some zealous practitioners have been seen to apply known beneficial techniques of "developmental stimulation" to sick infants with conditions that suggest the activity is counterindicated, causing needless pain, physiological stress, and medical risk.

Summary

Environmental stimulation in hospitals is inevitable, and the role of intentional stimulation programs for infants should be to assist in modifying the environment to provide adequate and appropriate developmental opportunities. Given the discomforts that are inherent with hospitalization and illness, maximizing comfort is of primary importance. For infants who are particularly at risk, maximizing their motivation as active learners and their parents' sense of competence and control, supersedes any other stimulation agenda. Reinforcing areas of health in the infant and the infant-family relationship should be a focus during the vulnerable time of hospitalization.

DISCUSSION

Frances Horowitz: Joy, is there any evidence that children receiving this kind of program in hospital recover more quickly, perhaps have fewer hospitalizations?

Joy Goldberger: I'm taking part in a grant at the moment to look at that question with three- to twelve-year-olds. I know of no research that addresses infants and toddlers in hospitals, but that's one of the projects that we're talking about doing next.

Arthur Parmelee: We've been interested in this for a long time, but you can imagine the logistics. Each child has a different disease, so we can't standardize it and demonstrate the shorter time for recovery. But clinically everybody is absolutely convinced—except the administration.

Cynthia Garcia Coll: It seems that the program is focused on the infant. What about the parents? How much input do the parents have?

Joy Goldberger: We support the position that parents know their child best, and we follow their lead and encourage parents as much as possible. We try to keep the family the most important thing that's happening for the infant. The challenge is maintaining involvement when parents find it hard to be available. I think things have gone full cycle. When I started nine years ago, very few parents were available and very few lived in. Living in wasn't fully encouraged and accepted yet. Over time parents increasingly started living in and being more available. And now there are more mothers in the work force and needing to go back to work to maintain the insurance that's paying for the hospitalization. There are also more young and single mothers with other young children. For the relatively brief stays of several days to a week, that is not too big an issue. Most of the parents can take vacation time for that. But for children with chronic health problems or hospitalized for extended stays, it's still a very big issue.

Peter Gorski: I'd like to thank you for so effectively reminding us of the patient's perspective, the child's perspective. Your discussion is very germane to the subject of preterm babies or high-risk infants who are hospitalized in NICUs (neonatal intensive care units). Increasingly now, neonates who are born very small and at highest risk grow up to be infants and even toddlers in our NICUs, because in many institutions we have no other facility able to care for these children, who require ongoing high-level medical support and yet begin to pass through stages of development while they are still in the hospital. And I have seen some breakthroughs in the physiological recovery process of babies only after the staff finally recognizes that this nine-month-old, for instance, or in another dramatic example a fifteen-month-old who had never left the hospital, was beginning to insist on exercising some autonomy about his life. The child had no control available to him, so the only way he could find was in very self-destructive ways of refusing to feed or holding his breath and turning blue when a physical therapy session was scheduled at the wrong time for him. Lots of examples like that occur in our daily experience. If we make sense of them, we can help the recovery process as well.

Joy Goldberger: One of the expressions we use is "making the most of what's healthy." We try to help parents make the most of their time with their infants. One of the things that we can do for parents is to remind them that while this system may be sick, there are still a lot of healthy systems there and that the child would much rather focus on what feels good and what's healthy. It can make a big difference all around.

Kathryn Barnard: For far too long we have all been dominated in hospital care by Parson's view of the illness role. He said that the individual must become dependent upon the health care provider and be separated from family, because if you separate from family you'll get well faster, because you'll want to go home. I think that's the antithesis to what we all know about the kind of security people need when they are ill. There are tremendous pressures on all health care providers now to contain costs, and so as you know, things like Child

Life programs are being cut out of hospital budgets. I think this is an opportunity for us to begin to emphasize the role of family members in the care of both children and adults in hospitals. We need to have familiar and secure people with us when we are ill or recovering. On the other hand, while it seems like a desirable goal, when you think about the employment situation of families where both parents are now working, it seems even more unachievable.

Peter Vietze: Joy, one of the things I was impressed with is the provision of a lot of visually responsive toys. What I missed was much attention to the auditory environment. If the one-minute contacts you talk about are typical, then babies in that situation must have a completely abnormal auditory language environment. I wondered what kinds of things you were doing there.

Joy Goldberger: That's probably the toughest thing. On the one hand we aim for each child's toys to include auditory and tactile as well as visual and motor benefits. On the other hand, the monitors are there, and the I-meds beeping, the radio, and all the other sounds. The best thing I know of for language is to keep the parents there. If you can keep the parents comfortable and help them feel welcomed and nonthreatened, then they are likely to be more relaxed and to be free to talk to their child. Scared parents probably talk less and are less responsive generally.

Also, my guess is that primary nurses who get involved with and attached to a patient are faster to respond to crying and other forms of communication than nurses who don't know their patients as well.

Arthur Parmelee: There's one problem that we ran into in providing a good many toys and pictures. Certain nurses and doctors seem to think that if the infants or children have these, they don't need much social interaction. We find we need to encourage social interactions and make sure they are not just a brief "hello." We put up a sign: "When you interact, stay 15 minutes or more."

Tiffany Field: Do they make use of foster grandmothers or volunteers?

Joy Goldberger: Selectively. In infancy the need for consistent people is so high that the foster grandparenting programs I like are the ones where one grandparent responds to one child, rather than ones where you have a grandparent each day of the week for whatever child needs it. I'm always concerned, however, that the parents might feel replaced.

I'm always an advocate for having Child Life on the unit, too, because Child Life specialists come with training in what to expect developmentally and emotionally and can provide supervision to such people as volunteers in grandparenting programs. Better yet, adequate Child Life staffing offers consistent caregivers and increases opportunities for attachment, predictable daily patterns, and developmentally appropriate play and encouragement, as well as therapeutic play.

ALLEVIATING STRESS IN ICU NEONATES

Tiffany Field, Ph.D.

Potentially stressful features of the neonatal intensive care unit (NICU), including continuous noise (Gottfried et al., 1981) and bright light (Glass et al., 1985), have recently generated concern among neonatal researchers. Some have speculated that the NICU may constitute an environment of sensory deprivation (Rothchild, 1966), while others have suggested that the preterm infant in the NICU may be overstimulated (Cornell & Gottfried, 1976) or may experience an inappropriate pattern of stimulation (Gottfried & Gaiter, 1985; Lawson, Daum, & Turkewitz, 1977). A recent volume on the NICU environment (Gottfried & Gaiter, 1985) suggests that there is little documented data on the effects of the NICU environment per se and even less data on the stressful effects of specific treatment procedures. This paper reviews the few studies that have examined the effects of stressful NICU procedures and reports on intervention studies designed to alleviate these stressful effects.

Stressful Procedures in the NICU

Long, Alistair, Philip, and Lucey (1980) found that increased heart rate and decreased $TcPO_2$ were associated with invasive procedures, such as heelsticks and intubation, and handling, such as during diaper changes. Personnel were instructed to use $TcPO_2$ monitoring to modify the care of low-birthweight infants and to limit procedures considered "undesirable time"—procedural time that contributed to reduced $TcPO_2$. When monitoring occurred, the amount of "undesirable time" was reduced from 40 minutes per 20 hours to 6 minutes per 20 hours. Infants in the monitored group were handled less frequently and experienced less hypoxemia.

More recently, other procedural stressors have been investigated, including the use of neurobehavioral assessments involving reflex testing and repositioning of the infant, as for example during the Brazelton Neonatal Behavioral Assessment Scale (NBAS), which is routinely conducted in many NICUs just prior to the preterm infant's discharge. Data from one study (Gunnar, Isensee, & Fust, in press) showed elevated cortisol levels following the administration of the NBAS, suggesting that assessments of this kind are stressful for the newborn. Although several neonatal researchers had noted behavioral distress in preterm neonates during and following the NBAS, this study was the first to document the stressful effects of neonatal assessments.

A physiological index of stress not previously used with preterm infants is growth hormone. While growth hormone levels are typically elevated in stressed adults and children, in stressed infants they are diminished (Stubbe & Wolf, 1971). A serendipitous finding in a study on the effects of stimulation (Schanberg & Field, in press) suggests that preterm neonates are also stressed by neurobehavioral assessments, as manifested by decreased growth hormone levels. In a sample of eight preterm infants, whose mean gestation age was 31 weeks and whose mean post-conceptional age was 36 weeks, growth hormone was found to drop an average of 32 percent between the day prior to the administration of the NBAS and two hours following its administration.

Findings like these have contributed to the "minimal touch" policies that have been adopted in many intensive care nurseries. They have also led to attempts to design shorter and less stressful neurobehavioral assessments for the preterm neonate (Als et al., 1982; Korner, 1986).

Being treated in an NICU and receiving routine procedures that are necessary for the survival and clinical well-being of the neonate also appear to be stressful. For example, heelsticks, necessary for bilirubin counts, have been reported to be associated with significant elevations in heart rate and respiration (Field & Goldson, 1984). In addition, weaning from mechanical ventilation has been found to be followed by elevated cortisol levels (Schanberg & Field, in press).

The Effects of Soothing Stimulation

To alleviate the general stress of being treated in an NICU and specific stress associated with those medical procedures that are necessary, researchers are exploring various forms of soothing stimulation that might be applied. Both natural caregiving stimulation, such as stroking the infant, and natural self-comforting behavior, such as sucking, appear to be helpful.

In one study designed to alleviate the general stress of being treated in an NICU, natural caregiving stimulation was given to very-short-gestation infants who required mechanical ventilation (Jay, 1982). Jay provided these infants 48 minutes of gentle tactile contact per day. A clinical nurse specialist simply placed her hands on the infant's head and abdomen for twelve minutes four times each day. The twelve-minute periods were planned around other activities so that they would not be interrupted. The objective was to provide the infant with periods of gentle touch during which the infant would not experience painful stimuli. This simple stimulation was associated with a decreased need for mechanical ventilation, fewer startle responses, and fewer clenched fists for the stimulated infants.

In a more extensive intervention (Field et al., 1986), preterm neonates were provided 45 minutes per day of stroking and passive movements of the limbs. The infants were recruited for the study at the time they entered the transitional "grower" nursery. The treatment group received tactile stimulation (stroking of the head and face region, neck and shoulders, back, legs, and arms) and kinesthetic stimulation (gentle flexing of the limbs) for three fifteen-minute periods during three consecutive hours per day for ten days. Clinical data recorded daily included formula intake and weight gain. At the end of the ten-day treatment period the Brazelton NBAS was administered, and each infant's sleep/wake behavior was recorded in a 45-minute observation period.

The results are summarized in Table 2. The stimulated infants averaged 47 percent greater weight gain per day than the control group, even though the groups did not differ in average formula intake. The treatment infants were awake and active a greater part of the behavioral observation period. The stimulated infants showed more mature habituation, orientation, motor activity, and range of state behavior on the NBAS. Finally, the infants in the treatment group were hospitalized for six fewer days than the control infants, yielding an average cost savings of $3,000 per infant. These studies suggest that simple forms of tactile stimulation can help to alleviate the general stress of being in an NICU and facilitate the clinical course of the preterm infant who has been treated in the NICU.

Table 2. Effects of Tactile-Kinesthetic Stimulation on Preterm Neonates

	Group		P
	Stimulation	**Control**	
Feedings (Mean number/day)	8.6	9.0	N.S.
Formula (Mean CCs/kg/day)	171.0	166.0	N.S.
Mean calories/kg/day	114.0	112.0	N.S.
Mean calories/day	169.0	165.0	N.S.
Daily weight gain (Mean grams)	25.0	17.0	.0005
Mean time awake	16.0%	7.0%	.04
Mean time in movement	32.0%	25.0%	.04
Mean Brazelton Scores			
Habituation	6.1	4.9	.02
Orientation	4.8	4.0	.02
Motor	4.7	4.2	.03
Range of State	4.6	3.9	.03

Source: Field et al., 1986

The infant can also apparently effectively modify stressful experiences with self-comforting behaviors such as sucking. In one study (Field & Goldson, 1984), NICU and minimal-care ("grower" nursery) preterm infants were given pacifiers during heelsticks. The infants who were allowed to suck on the pacifier during this stressful procedure showed less fussing and crying both during and after the procedure than those not given pacifiers (see Table 3). In addition, the more mature, minimal-care infants with pacifiers were less physiologically aroused by the procedure, as manifested by lower heart rates and respiration rates.

Table 3. Effect of Nonnutritive Sucking on Measures Taken
During Heelsticks in Minimal and Intensive Care Nurseries

| | Minimal Care | | | Intensive Care | | |
	Treatment	Control	P	Treatment	Control	P
Crying (Mean time)	25%	41%	.005	1%	19%	.001
Heart rate (Mean BPM)	172	187	.05	165	168	N.S.
Mean respiration rate	81	72	.05	51	54	N.S.

Source: Field & Goldson, 1984

Tube feeding is another stressful procedure during which nonnutritive sucking appears to calm the neonate. In a study by Field et al. (1982), neonates in the treatment group were given a pacifier during all tube feedings. The treatment group required fewer tube feedings than did the control group. Their average weight gain per day was also greater, they were hospitalized fewer days, and their hospital costs were significantly lower (see Table 4). In addition, infants in the treatment group were easier to feed during later bottle feedings. The nurses had to engage in fewer stimulating behaviors such as jiggling the bottle and changing the infant's position.

Table 4. Effects on Clinical Outcome Measures of Nonnutritive
Sucking During Tube Feedings

| | Group | | |
	Treatment	Control	P
Mean number of tube feedings	219.0	246.0	.05
Mean days of tube feeding	26.0	29.0	.01
Daily weight gain (Mean grams)	19.3	16.5	.05
Mean number of hospital days	48.0	56.0	.05
Mean hospital cost	$16,800.00	$20,294.00	.01

Source: Field et al., 1982

Summary

Natural caregiving stimulation such as gentle stroking and self-comforting stimulation such as sucking appear to attenuate distress behavior and physiology during stressful NICU procedures. These interventions are easy to provide, and given that they not only temporarily soothe the stressed infant but also have positive longer-term effects such as increased weight gain and shorter hospital stay, they would appear to be cost-effective means of alleviating stress for the NICU neonate.

DISCUSSION

Nico Spinelli: Harlow, in his work with mother-deprived infant monkeys, found that an amazing substitute for mother was a furry thing that they could cling to with belly contact. Since then we have been alerted to the fact that there are specific sensory stimuli that have disproportionate effects—I mean disproportionate from a naive point of view. Baby monkeys cling to the mother. Human babies don't do that. I'm wondering if the part that needs to be stroked the most is the one that would normally be in the best contact with the mother's body.

Tiffany Field: You mean the chest region. The problem is they don't like being massaged in that area, perhaps because many of the invasive procedures are performed on the chest region.

Berry Brazelton: In Colombia they send preemies home at two and three pounds if the mothers carry them between their breasts. Klaus and Kennell did a study there, and they became concerned that the babies were up against their mothers and would smother, and also that the babies ought to be looking out. So they tried them the other way, and the babies didn't gain weight and wouldn't tolerate it. They had to turn them back.

Barry Lester: What do you think is the meaning of these short-term changes in things like cortisol or growth hormone? How meaningful are they in terms of the levels that you're looking at and their potential implications? Do we have reason to be seriously concerned about these kinds of short-term changes?

Tiffany Field: I wouldn't be concerned about them. I just think it's important to know that they're there, and I like the idea of trying to modify any procedure, including the Brazelton Scale, that we're doing with the baby, on the basis of the baby's physiological reactions. Gunnar's data on cortisol elevations, if we can replicate these data, may suggest to the world that the NBAS may be a stressful procedure and that we should monitor the baby more closely while we're doing it, though I don't think we should throw it out. I think it's a temporary stress. I would doubt that if we went in three days later and looked at growth hormone levels they would still be depressed.

Kathryn Barnard: Tiffany, I was impressed that you said that from your observations so far it is the reflexes that are eliciting negative responses and that reflexes are really protective mechanisms. So if you are eliciting protective mechanisms, it seems reasonable that you are also activating other protective mechanisms, that the whole system may be activated, and that's why you get the decrease in growth hormone and increase in cortisol.

Also, a master's student of mine, Sandy Travatti, replicated Susan Jay's touching study as closely as she could. She also measured $TcPO_2$, heart rate, and respiration. What she found points to another possible interpretation of what the touching did. She found that there was essentially no change during, before, or after the touching in terms of $TcPO_2$ or heart rate, but over days the baby had more regular respiration during the touching period. It's as if the baby were beginning to learn some predictability about that touching experience, and it was helping regulate the whole respiratory problem.

Tiffany Field: That's what we've observed from their behaviors anecdotally. In the beginning they can feel us coming and they are aroused, and then over time they get very much into it.

Berry Brazelton: You should look at the growth hormone and the cortisol levels over time and see if there's learning that goes into it, an adaptation such as Bob was talking about.

Tiffany Field: We are. I've looked at some of our $TcPO_2$ data, which are on only a few babies so I don't really want to report these, but two out of the three babies showed slight elevations of $TcPO_2$ during the kinesthetic and not during the tactile stimulation, and one of the babies showed just the reverse. It occurred to me that this might be a way of determining which form of stimulation an individual infant prefers, because it seemed that, across the session, there was a nice pattern.

Cynthia Garcia Coll: There were some infants who did not show any weight gain with stimulation, and some who did. Did you find out anything about those babies, gestational age or anything, to account for this?

Tiffany Field: No, we looked very closely, because we were very concerned about those infants, and we couldn't find anything. The problem is that there are not enough of them to make any kind of statement.

Robert Isaacson: I'd like to respond to Berry's idea about looking at the corticosterone, or cortisol levels. Some years ago Bohus, Endroczi, and Lissak discovered that there was a much greater corticosterone response to the anticipation of a stressor than to the actual application of the stressor. This effect is substantial. There is about a threefold greater response to the anticipation of the stress experience than to the actual stress of the situation itself.

Edward Tronick: There are human data exactly on that by psychologists who have studied novice parachutists in the anticipation rather than at the jump.

Peter Vietze: Tiffany, have you looked at all at mother/infant interaction after discharge?

Tiffany Field: Not with this group. But if the baby is more responsive, as they appear to be on the Brazelton Scale, then the mother is inheriting a better baby at the end of the hospital period. And for that reason they may develop better interaction patterns.

Peter Vietze: That's an important question, then. There have been all sorts of attempts to make the babies more responsive, the assumption being that if the babies are more responsive the mothers will just grab them up. But that hasn't worked out very well in a lot of cases, and this might be a much more powerful stimulus for the mothers.

Anneliese Korner: Tiffany, I was as puzzled as you were about the results on many state observations. Could you tell me about when you were doing those observations—before the stimulation, or after? What's the time relationship?

Tiffany Field: We do observations during the stimulation and no-stimulation periods for two of those sessions—two days in the first week and two days in the second week—and then we have 45-minute sleep/wake observations that are separate, where there is no stimulation. Of course the reason we do the latter is to be able to compare the stimulated with the control group, because the stim/no-stim comparisons are within the stimulation group. They are generally consistent, though. They suggest that the stimulation is causing the babies to be more active.

Barry Nurcombe: It seems to me that state regulation is what is mediated by the effect of stroking. It seems likely to be hormonal as well. The question is, is it the stimulation of hormones which causes the metabolic effect?

Tiffany Field: I don't know whether it's hormonal or whether it's metabolic efficiency. There are studies that show that if malnourished children engage in more activity than they normally engage in, metabolic efficiency is significantly increased, and the weight gain is significant.

Barry Nurcombe: Surely this has to be a mediated effect; there has got to be something that comes in between. It must be hormonal. What else could it be? Magic?

PARADIGMS FOR INTERVENTION: INFANT STATE MODULATION

Kathryn E. Barnard, R.N., Ph.D.

Preterm infants show dysfunctional patterns of state modulation. During the early postnatal period they spend a large percentage of their time in an indeterminate sleep state, and as they mature their sleeping and awake states continue to differ from those of normal full-term infants.

Two experiments are described in this paper. In the first, a treatment was designed to help preterm infants organize sleep activity and have more quiet sleep during the incubator phase. The results from the neonatal period, a two-year follow-up, and an eight-year follow-up suggest positive influences on state organization and later cognitive functioning.

In the second experiment, infants in the post-incubator period were assisted in coming to a more alert state when awake. A strategy for bringing infants to a state of quiet alert prior to feeding has been shown to improve parent-infant interaction during feeding.

State Modulation in the Preterm Infant

An increasing challenge for the NICU (neonatal intensive care unit) health care provider is the type of environment that should be provided for the immature infant. I believe that the first issue is the infant's capacity for state modulation. Before considering any additional stimulation that may be helpful in promoting the infant's development, one should assist the infant in organizing within-state behavior and in making the transitions between states of sleep and wakefulness.

I see state modulation—the ability to get smoothly from one state to another and to maintain organization within a state—as the major developmental task of the neonate. State organization and modulation are seen in diurnal sleep patterns, a self-regulated feeding schedule, efficient feeding periods, and the ability to maintain alertness. State organization capacities are normally well differentiated by 44 weeks' gestational age, and by 52 weeks the ability to moderate cycles of sleep and activity is well patterned.

The preterm infant has more difficulty in state modulation than the full-term neonate. There are less well-organized states of sleep, wakefulness, and crying. As Dr. Parmelee has so well described (Garbanati & Parmelee, this volume), there is a lack of coherence in the biological systems, brain electrical activity, cardiovascular responses, and body movements. These individual physiological parameters mature at different rates and have different points in time when they begin to appear concurrently with other physiological subsystems.

In addition to the problem of state differentiation, the preterm infant experiences more difficulty in getting to sleep, in awakening, and in gaining a quality of alertness. Prior to 38 weeks' conceptional age, our priority is to help the infant organize sleep periods. After 40 weeks we can help them modulate periods of sleep and wakefulness, particularly functional alertness.

Structuring State Organization

The first example of environmental structuring we tried concerned sleep behaviors. This research grew out of my observations in the NICU. What was striking to me was that preterm infants did not seem able to inhibit their motion. They were in constant activity, much like the older hyperactive children we see with learning problems. These clinical observations motivated the effort to help preterm infants organize and maintain periods of quiet sleep.

In our first study (Barnard, 1973) we investigated the influence of a stimulation program in which the bed rocked gently while a heart beat tone was fed into the incubator. Infants in the experimental program were found to have an increase in the amount of quiet sleep and a more rapid weight gain than the control group. In a later study (Barnard & Bee, 1983), temporally patterned stimulation with a rocker-bed and heart beat tone was tested on infants born prior to 35 weeks' gestational age. Three experimental variations of stimulation were used: fixed interval (infants received fifteen minutes of stimulation every hour), self-activating (infants received fifteen minutes of stimulation after remaining quiet for 90 seconds), and quasi-self-activating (infants received 15 minutes of stimulation after 90 seconds of inactivity, but only for one stimulation period per hour). All experimental infants as compared with controls showed decreased rates of activity while in the hospital, shorter and thus increased activity cycles, fewer abnormal reflexes, better orienting responses, better state regulation, and higher scores on the Bayley Mental Development Index (MDI) at 24 months. Infants in the quasi-self-activating group were consistently above those in the other two experimental groups on measures that showed a difference.

The treatment groups had differences in the amount of stimulation. The self-activating group had almost twice as much stimulation per day as the others, and they were on it a longer time than the others. For these infants there was a reduction of body activity and eye movement during the period of stimulation. For the other two groups, which had a fixed interval component, the reduction of body activity came not so much during the rocking period as during the five-minute period after it. For these infants, it seemed as though the eye movement characteristic of active or transitional sleep was suppressed during the stimulation. When the stimuli went off, the result was a burst of eye movement and a reduction of body movement.

In spite of these differences in the amount of stimulation and in reaction to stimulation, there were no other striking differences between the treatment groups during the hospital period or at two years that could be related to these stimulation differences. The clinical course of the infants did not vary for the treatment and control groups. A surprising finding was that no differences were found in parent-infant interaction during the early neonatal period or later during the first year of life. Spontaneous reports from the nursing staff that the treatment babies were easier to feed had led us to expect such differences, but the infants in the later study were no more alert and responsive during feeding than the control infants.

At 24 months we again looked at parent-child interaction, and this time there was one item in which there was a difference. We asked the mothers to teach the children something, and during a hard task the fixed-interval-group mothers tended to give more negative messages to the children, while the self-activated-group mothers gave the least negative feedback. On the Bayley MDI, the treatment groups looked better, with the quasi-self-activated group scoring highest. Those infants had both the experience of contingency in turning the rocker on and a discrimination learning task in learning when they could turn the bed on and when they couldn't. We also found that on Bettye Caldwell's HOME (Home Observation for Measurement of the Environment) Inventory the treatment group had higher scores on two subscales: the organization of the environment by the mother and the variety of daily stimulation.

We have just completed our eight-year follow-up and found that the treatment group had higher scores on the WISC (Wechsler Intelligence Scale for Children) and the Beery Test of Visual-motor Integration. The self-activating group had the best score on the Beery test. We are now questioning whether it was the more stimulation the self-activating group had or the fact that the stimulation was contingent. We are still checking our results, and these should be considered preliminary, unconfirmed trends.

Increasing Alertness

An equally important task for the infant is to develop increasing control over the occurrence and quality of awake periods. An important influence on the development of the preterm infant's ability to regulate and modulate levels of arousal is the interaction between the infant and caregivers. Caregiving, especially when related to feeding, has been demonstrated to be associated with significant state modulation and the development of 24-hour rhythms in the preterm infant (Blackburn & Barnard, 1985; Blackburn, 1978).

By the time they come home from the hospital, most preterm infants are well enough entrained to a three- to four-hour feeding schedule that they come to a semi-arousal at these periods. The quality of the infant's alertness at these times, however, is less than optimal. Parents describe feeding periods that last over an hour, with the baby alternately sucking briefly and falling into sleepiness. Several studies comparing preterm and full-term infants on the Brazelton Scale (Telzrow et al., 1982; Kang & Barnard, 1979; Barnard, 1980) have confirmed this clinical observation, finding preterm infants to have a lower level of behavioral responsiveness.

In a more recent study, we compared mother-infant interaction with term and preterm infants considered at high risk socially because of low maternal education and income. We found that the preterm infants had less desirable interaction in the feeding observation at three months. We therefore developed an intervention to influence directly the quality of alertness prior to a feeding. The parents are taught to recognize the different states of sleep and wakefulness and to learn how to help the infant increase the level of functional alertness. We teach the principle of providing a varied pattern of stimuli for arousal and repetitious patterning for soothing. We also alert them to the behavioral signs of overload, such as color changes, state lowering, and irritability. We show them how to go through some gentle procedures of stroking, undressing, talking, and cuddling the baby for ten to fifteen minutes before feeding, to get the baby to a nice state of quiet alert.

In the first test of this feeding treatment (Fuhrmann, 1984), infants in the experimental group had significantly higher scores than controls on the Nursing Child Assessment Feeding Scales, and all feedings took less than thirty minutes. The interaction score was positively correlated with the infant's alertness prior to feeding.

We have subsequently replicated these findings in a field trial with a larger sample (Barnard et al., 1987). We found that the babies who had the state modulation feeding treatment scored higher than their counterpart terms at the same living age and a significantly higher score than term babies at the same adjusted or conceptional age. Moreover, these benefits continued, for both infants and mothers. Mothers who were helped to learn how to alert their infants before feeding do not show the burnout that we have seen in some other studies.

DISCUSSION

Barry Lester: Your eight-year follow-up brings up the notion of sleeper effects. I was wondering if you had any thoughts about how you might interpret it.

Kathryn Barnard: I am impressed with the exquisite ability of the young infant to take in the environment. At every level, the infant is so sensitive to the environment that the things I worry most about are those that provide a consistent long-term pattern. I think those are the types of experiences that are probably going to have the most profound impact. If something lasts only for a little while you probably don't really need to worry about having either positive or negative results. But in those early experiences that set off some kind of chain, either in the environment/infant interaction or in the infant/parent interaction, then I think there is the possibility for either harm or good.

We've seen one interesting thing, and I have no idea what this means. We began to have the parents in the study come in for parents' groups, because as we followed them up we found them very anxious about whether their children were going to develop problems as a result of their prematurity. During the group sessions, I had college students in psychology watching the children and the siblings. I would debrief them, and the thing that struck me consistently was that they would describe the children who were treatment subjects—they didn't know who was treatment and who was control—as being more social and less clumsy. Until we got this eight-year result with the Beery and some of the performance scales, I never really thought that there might be something to that. One of the problems concerning these earlier experiences is that we don't really understand all the pathways that may be mediated.

Nico Spinelli: The cats in our study are also different, even though they spend most of their time playing around being cats. They are noticeably more alert and more attentive. It seems to me that there are two types of early experiences. There is the constant deluge of all sorts of meaningless stimuli, and then there are those experiences that have triggering effects and that are seminal to what will happen later. It strikes me that your rocking bed has tremendous parallels with what we do. There is a clear action effect in which causality is neatly working. Normally children, not to mention kittens, have to discover causality and this chain of actions by extracting them from the noise of all sorts of things that are going on all the time. This archetypical experience, I think, serves as a blueprint for many other similar experiences later on in which the organism learns very quickly that there is a pattern of action. You do something, you expect something. This may seem simple to us, but I think it's such a momentous happening at that time that from then on it can have a really substantive effect.

Berry Brazelton: This is all certainly true of burned children. The literature on recovery from burns shows that as soon as you give the child something that he can act on and get feedback from he begins to improve significantly.

Peter Vietze: Kathy, basically you were giving a learning study. When did the infants show evidence of learning to control the bed?

Kathryn Barnard: Well, they turned it on a lot.

Peter Vietze: Yes, but when we look at contingent control, we can evaluate whether they learned or not.

Kathryn Barnard: I think they learned, because the amount of time they had the bed turned on increased over time.

Peter Vietze: There have been some analyses of young babies' abilities to learn in operant fashion, which basically this was. And some people suggest that newborns don't have the memory capacity to learn. John Watson did a fairly elegant analysis a long time ago showing that it's roughly around eight weeks when babies begin to be able to remember long enough to link the behavior and the reinforcing stimulus, and these would be interesting data to study.

Kathryn Barnard: Some of these babies had the rocker bed on twenty-two times a day or more, so they had very repetitive experiences with contingency.

Craig Ramey: Did you say that there were some differences in activity levels of the children?

Kathryn Barnard: In the nursery.

Craig Ramey: How about later? One of the plausible mechanisms—and we have some evidence for this in some of our research—is that the function of intervention is to change the child's propensity to engage. It doesn't necessarily change the responsivity of the mother. Her responsivity will increase as a conditional probability. She doesn't respond any more frequently, but because the child makes more bids, the child ends up getting more feedback. So activity might be a mediating variable that would lead to some of these differences.

Kathryn Barnard: We probably haven't looked at initiations as carefully as you have with the child, but on any activity measure that we've done in terms of parent-child interaction we don't see any differences.

Peter Gorski: Kathy, I'm curious if there is any separate effect of the heart tone. I don't remember if you unlinked that.

Kathryn Barnard: No, we didn't, but that would be interesting to do.

PARENTAL STIMULATION OF HIGH-RISK INFANTS IN NATURALISTIC SETTINGS

Peter M. Vietze, Ph.D.

Experimental evidence accumulated over the years has helped to define how infant stimulation facilitates infant development. Recent advances in technology have led to greater success in saving very small and very sick neonates. These tiny infants must stay in the neonatal intensive care unit (NICU) for weeks, often months, and thus are separated from their parents for long periods during a stage when parents, especially mothers, are thought to provide significant stimulation to their infants. Nevertheless, we are not sure what constitutes optimal stimulation for infants in NICUs. In fact, it is not clear that we can define criteria for optimal maternal stimulation for any infant.

This paper attempts to define some criteria for optimal maternal stimulation of infants, especially in the domain of vocalization. It draws on research on several longitudinal samples, including normal middle-income infants, normal and high-risk lower-income infants, and infants with Down's syndrome, and on a cross-sectional study of handicapped infants.

The Research Design

Our first task was to design an observational instrument that we could use to characterize mother-infant interaction. We wanted to capture the quality, variety, and timing of each partner's behavior as they conducted their business. We were most interested in understanding the contingencies in the interaction, especially whether and how mothers responded contingently to their infants. After experimenting with various approaches, we settled on a technique that preserved the sequence and pattern of mother and infant behavior and allowed maximum flexibility in coding and analysis. The studies reported here all utilized this observational system to collect data.

The observational system (Anderson et al., 1978) consisted of a set of numerical codes representing patterns of infant and mother behavior. Each behavior pattern is defined as a composite of one or more behavior categories. For infants, there are five behavior categories: (1) visual attention to mother, (2) nondistress vocalization, (3) smile, (4) distress vocalization (crying), and (5) no signalling behavior present ("none"). Similarly, five behavioral categories are recorded for the mother: (1) visual attention to the infant, (2) vocalization directed to the infant, (3) smile, (4) tactile play stimulation, and (5) no behavior directed to the infant. Thus one maternal behavior pattern would be looking at the infant while vocalizing and smiling. In addition to codes for each behavior pattern observed, codes were also entered for the contexts of infant arousal state, maternal proximity to the infant, and maternal caregiving activities.

Observational data were treated in two ways. First, we aggregated the data to determine the total duration of visual attention, vocalization, smiling, touch-playing, and "none" as well as the different levels of the three contexts. This aggregation was made by summing the individual behaviors from the patterns which were observed to make categories. The patterns indicate what actually happened, while the categories summarize each behavior from the patterns. Second, since we were interested in contingent interactional behaviors, we also subjected the data to time-series analysis, using the method described by Stern (1974), Anderson and Vietze (1977), and Bakeman and Brown (1977).

Study 1. Normal Middle-Income Families

This study was a baseline investigation of 49 normal middle-income infants and mothers observed in their homes when the infants were 2 1/2, 6 1/2, and 12 1/2 months of age. Observations were conducted at a time when the infant was judged to be alert and awake and included a feeding time and a play time.

Over the course of the three observations, infant behavior showed developmental changes, with the pattern of vocalizing alone increasing and visual attention alone decreasing. "None" and crying also decreased with age.

The mothers' behavior patterns showed little change as the infant grows older, although when the data are aggregated by category there seems to be a trend toward decreasing vocalizing and visual attention between 2 1/2 and 6 1/2 months and for smiling between 6 1/2 and 12 1/2 months.

These are individual behavior measures for each partner taken during a dyadic examination. In order to derive dyadic measures, we had to construct variables in which both partners' behavior was taken into account. We therefore classified the dyad's behavior at each instance of observation according to one of four states: (1) mother behaving, infant not behaving; (2) infant behaving, mother not behaving; (3) both behaving; and (4) neither behaving. The behavior record now looked like a chain of the sequence of these four states.

The next step was to classify the sequential chain according to the transitions from one state to the next. Since we were interested in evaluating the responsiveness of the mother to the infant, we focused on some specific comparisons. The model for maternal responsivity is that the infant does something and the mother responds soon afterward. Because vocal behavior was considered extremely important for development, the analyses were carried out only on vocal behaviors emitted by mother and infant. Thus the behavior pattern that reflected maternal responsiveness was the transition from infant vocalizing (IV) to both vocalizing (BV)—that is, the mother joining the infant in vocalizing. This was our operational definition of maternal vocal responsiveness, or maternal contingent vocalization.

In order to evaluate whether the mother's vocal responsiveness changed with the infant's increasing age, we compared the transition IV to BV with a measure of the mother's tendency to vocalize when the infant was not vocalizing, NV to MV. We found that the mother's base rate of initiating vocalization did not change over the first year, but her contingent vocalization did. Between 2 1/2 and 6 1/2 months it declined somewhat, and it then increased between 6 1/2 and 12 1/2 months.

Study 2. Mentally Retarded Infants

This was a cross-sectional study of children who were generally functioning at the level of twelve-month-olds but whose average age was 29 months. There were 26 infants with various degrees of disability and with various etiologies, including Down's syndrome, perinatal casualty, microcephaly, and other less specific diagnoses. The observations were conducted in the homes using the same observational instrument as in the previous study. In order to determine whether mother-infant interaction was affected by developmental levels, the group was divided according to mental age (M.A.) as measured by the Bayley Scales.

In most of the infant behavior patterns, the different developmental levels conformed to the age differences in the normal sample. Thus, the high M.A. children showed more vocalization and less looking than the low M.A. children. Their mothers also showed behavior similar to the mothers of the normal children. There was not much evidence of the mothers adjusting their behavior patterns according to the developmental level of their children. When we examined the aggregates of the separate categories, however, we found more evidence that the mothers accommodated to the changing developmental level of the infants, with the mothers of the high M.A. children exhibiting more looking, smiling, and touch-playing and less vocalization than the mothers of low M.A. children. Thus, as the infants become more vocal, the mothers are probably talking less overall and allowing the infants to talk more. We shall see how this works when we discuss the sequential analysis below.

The sequential analysis showed that the mothers of high M.A. children showed less contingent responding and less vocalization in general. But the contingent responding drops more relative to the mother's vocal output. The infant contingent vocalization is similar for the handicapped children as for the normal children. Finally, there is some evidence that the higher functioning retarded children are less likely to stop vocalizing contingent on the mother's vocalization, but there is not much difference in the two developmental levels. In general, there is less tendency to cease vocalization in the high M.A. group. In the normal sample, the tendency to cease vocalization drops sharply but only until six months.

Study 3. Low-Income, Low-Birthweight Infants

These data are derived from a prospective longitudinal study of low-income families designed to predict child abuse, nonorganic failure to thrive, and neglect (Altemeier et al., 1979). A group of 598 infants and mothers was followed from pregnancy to twelve months. As part of the study, infants with birthweights under 2,500 grams were compared with those from Study 1, using the interaction system described above. The mothers and infants were observed at birth in the hospital and when the infant was one, three, six, and twelve months of age.

Infant vocalization increased over the first year, as it did for normal middle-class children, but the trend is erratic, not the smooth developmental trend seen for the normal children. The "none" category decreases with age and is higher than for the normal children or the handicapped children. Visual attention increases with age, rather than decreasing.

What about the mothers? These mothers show extremely low rates of vocalization—much lower than that for the mothers of the normal middle-class children or the mothers of the handicapped children (whose high rate may have been the result of their participation in early intervention). Maternal contingent vocalization is high during the newborn period, however, then declining to below the level for the other two groups. These mothers seem to be overstimulating their infants as newborns and understimulating them after the first month.

It would seem, then, that the mothers of low-birthweight infants need to be taught ways to provide appropriate contingent stimulation to enhance the infant's vocal production. What is the best way to do this? The next study will provide some clues.

Study 4. Mother-Infant Interaction in Infants with Down's Syndrome

In this study (McQuiston, 1982) mothers and infants came to our laboratory and were videotaped during spontaneous free play, a brief still-face period, and a period during which the mother was asked to imitate her infant. The study included eleven Down's syndrome infants and eleven nonhandicapped infants.

Data from the study confirm the frequent observation that mothers of Down's syndrome infants emit high rates of behavior when interacting with their babies. This may be why the rates of infant vocalization were much lower in this group than in the control group during spontaneous play at three months. Infants learn early to take turns in conversation. If the mothers of Down's syndrome infants are extremely active, their infants' vocal production will be low. In the imitation condition, the Down's syndrome infants almost treble their vocal output; normal infants increased less. In imitating, the Down's syndrome mothers had to slow down, watch carefully and produce a matching response, allowing the infant to increase vocal output and experience contingent feedback. At six months both groups showed dramatic increases between the two conditions. Perhaps their mothers had used this strategy during the three months between observations. The data on smiling suggest that the mothers of Down's syndrome infants engage in excessive smiling in order to elicit smiling from their infants—perhaps to make the child feel more like a person to them. Under the imitation condition, smiling is reduced for both groups.

Intervention Strategies

The lessons from these studies are brief. Adult caregivers interacting with infants must wait for the infant to act before responding, especially in the vocal modality, if the infant is to be given a chance to become social. Imitating teaches adult caregivers to be sensitive to the infant's behavior, allows the infant to pace the interaction, and provides contingent feedback that will build the infant's repertoire.

DISCUSSION

Kathryn Barnard: Peter, we have some interesting data from a master's student, Marian Morio. She looked at the episodes of verbal behavior during the first year of life in 27 mother-infant pairs and then at the episodes of pauses. At about eight months the mothers doubled the length of their pauses, as though they were waiting for the infant to initiate the response.

Nico Spinelli: It always amazes me that evolution has not built into the genes, so to speak, the perfect mother. There is so much learning to be done about being a mother. That seems to suggest that being a good mother takes the environment into consideration. Are there some aspects of being a mother that are not environmentally dependent and some that are?

Peter Vietze: First of all, I don't agree with you that it's not built in.

Nico Spinelli: A big piece is built in, but then there is a lot to be learned. So what is the built-in part, and what is the part that needs to be learned?

Peter Vietze: Perhaps some details about looking at the baby, paying attention to the baby rather than performing some caregiving activity, may be learned. And that different ways of paying attention may have different effects in different environments. We sometimes see examples of mothers' attention-giving that seem intrusive. This intrusiveness may be the result of our psychologizing to mothers in this country. There's a lot written about what you should do with babies. Titles of books suggest "Stimulate Your Baby" or "Teach Your Baby," and that may not be the best advice. When mothers are being intrusive, they are doing what they think is expected rather than following their own intuition. With a normal baby, the mother's instinctive way of responding is probably the best way. And I think that one of the problems that occur when a baby is labeled somehow is that the mother begins to short-circuit her natural tendency, her instinct.

Joy Goldberger: I see that in mothers of babies who may have been sick but were developmentally pretty much intact. Someone has taught the mother just what she should do, and she comes to me and asks, "Now what do I do?" And these are mothers who probably would have done just fine, who would have known what to do. They have to learn to trust their instincts.

Edward Tronick: Many mothers today do not have the social support systems through which women used to learn parenting. I think use of words like intuition and instinct mask the possibility that the mother has missed certain kinds of learning experiences that in the past would have allowed that kind of learning to take place. That's one reason why we may need to teach something as fundamental as parenting. We've distorted the early developmental process in a lot of ways. Another way is by writing too much and having well-educated mothers read too much. The process is also distorted by the kind of children we're talking about. High-risk and preterm infants did not have to be dealt with formerly.

Also, just as we talk about the stages of development, we can talk about stages of parenting, and the initial stage should probably be thought of as a hazard-prevention strategy. In order to do that in different ecologies, because humans exist in different ecologies, you need a lot of flexibility in the system to make those adjustments. And those patterns are culturally based patterns. In our society, we're compromising the parents because of cultural problems.

Cynthia Garcia Coll: A lot of the cultural pockets that we have in the United States still have the extended family from which mothers learn. The U.S. is very heterogeneous in terms of social class, ethnic background, and some traditions about parenting, and sometimes I find myself hesitating about teaching some mothers who are accustomed to looking to a family member for guidance. We have to be very sensitive to those ethnic differences.

Edward Tronick: In discussing his data on the cat, Nico talked about surprise, and a number of times since then we've talked about special experiences, or triggering experiences. I thought a really critical point is that with the cat the quantity of experience that the animal had with the contingency in the environment really didn't matter. It was very small. I think the same point was made in some of your results, Jennifer, where you got that differentiation based on the probability of events. And here you're talking about key critical kinds of experiences, Peter. Is there some dimension other than quantity we need to think about, like the information about surprise or contingency?

Peter Vietze: In a number of our studies we monitored visual attention to the stimulus that was made contingent on the infant's responding. We found that a repetitive, non-response-dependent, so-called noncontingent stimulus is habituated; the infant stops looking at it. A contingent stimulus, on the other hand, is variable. In addition to the baby's having control over it, it varies in temporal sequence and patterning and it's a much richer kind of stimulus. The baby attends to it much longer.

Also, I mentioned that smiling is at a low level. We were very disappointed in that, because the dominant white middle-class culture puts a lot of stock in smiling, and psychoanalytic literature thinks that smiling is very important. It carries affect, it carries a lot of meaning, and yet it doesn't occur much. The fact that it doesn't occur more often may give it its information value when it does occur. In the same way, in traditional homes where the father goes out and works and the mother stays home, the father seems to have some extra information value. He's more of a surprising stimulus, because he's not there as much. The mother is taken for granted. She may be there all the time, and the baby habituates.

THE MOTHER-INFANT TRANSACTION PROGRAM: AN INTERVENTION FOR THE MOTHERS OF LOW-BIRTHWEIGHT INFANTS

Virginia A. Rauh, Sc.D.,
Barry Nurcombe, M.D., F.R.A.C.P.,
Thomas Achenbach, Ph.D.,
and Catherine Howell, Ph.D.

The low-birthweight (LBW) infant expends so much energy maintaining the homeostasis of blood flow, respiration, and temperature that little may be left for social interaction. The preterm infant's immature nervous system tends to become overloaded or exhausted. His unstable control of state allows little if any of the quiet alertness that is the most favorable time for productive social interaction. In sum, the preterm infant tends to be poorly regulated, unpredictable, and inaccessible.

From the parent's perspective, the infant is likely to be aversive in size and skin color. He is barricaded behind technical devices, his survival or ultimate integrity in doubt. The mother may be in the throes of an emotional crisis caused by the premature birth.

Despite these hazards, if birthweight is not exceptionally low, and provided there is no gross damage to the infant's central nervous system, the best predictor of later development is the socioeconomic status (SES) of the parents. The implication is that, except in extreme conditions, effective parenting can overcome the biological adversity of premature birth. By the same token, the parent encumbered by poverty, poor social support, mental illness, personality disorder, or defective emotional experiences in her own childhood may be unable to compensate for the LBW infant's neurophysiological handicaps. The stage is then set for progressively less favorable mother-infant transactions, which compromise both the infant's development and the parents' adjustment (Sameroff & Chandler, 1975).

Theoretically, it might be possible to intervene to forestall the downward spiral of unfavorable transactions. Such an intervention would need to be undertaken early, before an adverse pattern of interaction had become established, yet not so early that the mother would not be able psychologically to profit from it. It would also have to be economically feasible—neither unduly protracted nor excessively extravagant in staff requirements.

The Vermont Mother-Infant Transaction Program (MITP) was designed with both economy and feasibility in mind. Implemented by a specially trained neonatal intensive care nurse, the MITP consisted of seven daily sessions conducted during the week prior to the infant's discharge from the hospital and four subsequent sessions conducted in the home three, fourteen, thirty, and ninety days following discharge. Whenever possible, fathers were also involved.

Subjects in the study included 78 LBW infants (less than 2,250 grams and gestational age under 37 weeks), who were assigned by the toss of a coin to LBW Intervention (N=38) and LBW Control (N=40) groups. An additional comparison group consisted of 41 full-term, normal-birthweight infants (NBW).

Aims of the Intervention

1. To enable the mother to appreciate her infant's unique characteristics, temperament, and developmental potential.

2. To sensitize the mother to the infant's cues, particularly those signalling stimulus overload or exhaustion and those indicating a state conducive to interaction.

3. To teach the mother to respond appropriately and in timely fashion to infant cues indicating overload, distress, exhaustion, or readiness for interaction.

4. To enable the mother to embed her sensitivity and contingent responsiveness in the everyday tasks of cleaning, bathing, dressing, feeding, and soothing the infant.

5. To enhance the mother's enjoyment of her baby.

No direct attempt was made to supply "compensatory stimulation." Ultimately, the MITP aimed to promote dyadic reciprocity by modeling skills, providing verbal instruction and direct demonstration, offering emotional support when appropriate, and reinforcing the mother's own initiative

Schedule of Intervention

Day 1. Introduction. The first session was used to become acquainted with the mother, to explain the intervention, and to demonstrate the infant's uniqueness and potential for self-regulation and interaction. The nurse first conducted the Brazelton Neonatal Behavorial Assessment. She then explored the mother's perceptions of the baby and her experiences with the baby. The mother was encouraged to discuss the reactions of her husband and family to the baby and any fears about the future. If the baby fell short of her ideal, the nurse helped her to perceive his special qualities.

Day 2. Homeostasis. Signs of infant distress, disorganization, and exhaustion were examined and distinguished from signs of composure and stability. Sources of environmental stress were discussed, such as cold, loud noise, bright light, or sudden movement, and indices of homeostatic breakdown were presented (see Table 5). The mother analyzed the environmental stresses to which her infant was most sensitive and learned how to support his homeostatic controls by providing warmth, moderate lighting, soothing sounds, and gentle, rhythmic movements.

Day 3. The motor system. The nurse introduced the concept that posture, tone, and movement can signal disorganization, and the mother learned to discriminate smooth from jerky movements, abrupt from gradual alterations of muscle tone, and undifferentiated body movements from well-modulated movements of hands, arms, and legs (see Table 6). The nurse demonstrated how the infant could inhibit his own startles, twitches, and tremors and how the caregiver could aid the infant to do so.

Table 5. Homeostatic Systems in the Excited Infant and the Well-Organized Infant

System	Excited Infant	Well-Organized Infant
Respiration	Irregularity Apnea	Smooth, regular respiration
Skin circulation	Harlequin syndrome Cyanosis Paleness Flushing or mottling	Good, even, healthy color
Automatically mediated movement	Frequent tremors or startles	Few spontaneous tremors or startles
Facial movement	Twitches and automatic eye movements (rolling and floating)	Few, except normal mouthing, sucking, and grimacing
Visceral activity	Whimpering Hiccoughing Spitting up Gagging Grunting Bowel movement straining	Few visceral cues except mild sighing

Intervention continued to emphasize that the baby's behavior could be an index to his level of organization, and gradually the mother learned to respond to his cues in ways that allayed distress and promoted organization.

Day 4. State regulation. The nurse demonstrated the levels of sleep, drowsiness, alertness, and fussing, reviewing how these levels could be recognized by their autonomic and motoric characteristics, and showed how the infant responded differently at each level. Together, nurse and mother noted the baby's predominating states and worked on how to recognize and take advantage of the quiet alertness state.

The nurse also demonstrated how the baby regulated himself, and the mother was encouraged to experiment with ways of helping him organize himself when he was distressed.

Table 6. Motor Systems in the Excited Infant and the Well-Organized Infant

System	Excited Infant	Well-Organized Infant

Posture	Hyperextension
	Hyperflexion
	Flaccidity
	Abrupt alterations
	Lack of postural
	  adjustment
		Consistent smoothness
		  and modulation

Tone	Hypertonicity
	Hypotonicity
	Abrupt alterations
	Lack of tonal
	  adjustment
		Good, consistent,
		  modulated tone
		  throughout body

Movement	Jerky movements of
	  legs and arms
	Frantic, diffuse activity
	  alternating with no
	  activity at all
	Undifferentiated whole
	  arm and leg
	  movements
	Lack of activity
		Smooth, well-
		  modulated movement
		  of head and extremities

Day 5. Social interaction. The mother learned how to engage the infant and sustain social interaction with him. She learned how to recognize when he would be responsive to social interaction and how to sustain his alertness with animate and inanimate stimuli, at the same time remaining attentive to signals of impending overstimulation.

Day 6. Daily care. The mother was now ready to provide daily care in a more effective manner. She learned to coordinate daily activities with the infant's cycles of arousal and sleep and to embed her enhanced sensitivity and responsiveness in daily caretaking (see Table 7).

Day 7. Preparing for home. The previous six days were reviewed. The mother practiced alerting and enjoying her baby. The nurse encouraged her to use her new knowledge and trust her own initiative about how to alert, engage, and support her baby. Finally, the nurse explained that the domestic situation would make new demands on infant and parents and that a period of adjustment would be required.

Table 7. Daily Activities with the Easily Stressed Infant

Activity	Techniques
Waking	Enter room slowly, turn on light, and open curtains slowly. Vocalize softly. Uncover or unwrap infant gradually. Avoid overstimulating, even if infant is difficult to arouse.
Changing	Adjust room temperature. Avoid sudden changes in infant's position. Contain infant's limbs while shifting position. Keep tactile stimulation very mild. Frequent consoling may be necessary, but allow baby to exert self-quieting mechanisms.
Feeding	Attend to infant's unique demands for feeding. Time feeding to coincide with spontaneous alert periods. Avoid inessential noise. Inhibit disorganized motor activity by wrapping infant or holding him close to body. Adjust distance from caregiver to suit infant.
Bathing	As above, proceed slowly, watching for signs of exhaustion and disrganization (tremor, pallor, flailing, limpness). Ventral openness may be disruptive. Ventral body surface inhibition may be needed, using hands or feet against hand or bedside. Cover body parts not being washed. Offer support as needed in the form of a finger or pacifier. Allow frequent rests. Allow infant to organize himself rather than attempting to console him.

Home visit 1 (day 3 at home). Consolidation. The nurse reviewed with the parents the adjustment of everyone to the domestic situation. She ascertained whether the mother's sensitivity to, responsiveness to, and enjoyment of her baby had deteriorated, and if so she encouraged the mother to discuss problems. The nurse then helped the mother to define her own style of responding, in order to explore how well it matched the baby's style of response. The nurse identified the mother's strengths, reinforcing them and supporting her confidence in her own initiative.

Home visit 2 (two weeks at home). Mutual enjoyment through play. By now, infant and parents were better adjusted. Mutually accommodated and attuned, mother and infant would have more time for social interaction. The nurse reinforced the exploration of new opportunities and new media for play. Nurse and mother noted which activities the parents and the infant found most rewarding, and the nurse suggested a variety of techniques to help the parents expand their repertoire (see Table 8).

Home visit 3 (one month at home). Temperamental patterns. The purpose of this visit was to introduce the mother to the concept of infant temperament. The mother was helped to discern the infant's emerging response style (see Table 9) and to appreciate the effect of his temperament on their interaction. She learned that she could enhance the "fit" between the infant and herself by taking into consideration her baby's likes and dislikes. If the mother was frustrated and discouraged, the nurse helped her express her concerns.

Final home visit (three months at home). Review and termination. The nurse reviewed with the mother the autonomic, homeostatic and motor reflex systems. Current skin color, respiratory regulation, vocalization, facial expression, posture, tone, and movement were evaluated. By this time, the infant was usually more stable physiologically and better controlled motorically. Since the communicative skills of the infant were still rudimentary, however, it was essential for the parent to remain responsive to his physical cues.

The nurse assessed the infant's visual, auditory, and tactile development, asking the mother to recall recent progress. The mother was encouraged to trace the evolution of the infant's cycle of sleep and waking.

The results of the intervention were reviewed. To what degree had parental knowledge, sensitivity, responsiveness, caregiving skill, and mutual enjoyment been promoted? To the extent that these goals had been achieved, the parents would be ready to progress to challenging the infant in more advanced play.

At the end of the final session, the parents were presented with a photograph of their baby and a logbook of the baby's development as perceived by the nurse in each intervention session.

Table 8. Methods of Initiating Play

Sensory Channel	Play Modalities
Visual	Recognize periods of alertness.
	Engage the infant visually, using facial stimulation.
	Sustain eye-to-eye contact.
	Change your facial expression in order to sustain visual interaction, using smiling, expressions of surprise, tongue movements.
	Move your head, encouraging infant to follow.
	Move, nod, and shake your head to sustain the interaction.
	Imitate the infant's facial expressions.
	Use bright objects to help the infant focus and follow.
	Hold the infant upright so he can see over your shoulder.
	Position the infant's seat so he can watch you.
Auditory	Appreciate that the infant can attend to a variety of sounds.
	Use your voice in a variety of ways to communicate with the infant (singing, humming, clucking, calling name, talking).
	Attempt to get the infant to turn his eyes and head toward your voice.
	Imitate the infant's vocalizations.
	Use inanimate objects to make new sounds for the infant to hear (rattles, bells, music).
Tactile	Attempt to keep infant organized during periods of alertness, using wrapping, hand-holding, holding, positioning.
	Touch, pat, and stroke the infant in a soothing and rhythmical manner.
	Use the infant's reflex behavior to stimulate movement and contact (e.g., rooting leads to sucking; a finger inserted into a fist is grasped).
	Hold and cuddle the infant.
	Rock the infant when he is quiet, and console him by rocking when he fusses.
	Move around with the infant upright against your shoulder.
	Combine body and facial movement by kissing and nuzzling the infant.
	Imbed playful contact in instrumental tasks such as changing and bathing.

Table 9. Behavioral Cues to Infant Temperament

Dimension	Behavior
Activity level	Motor activity and sleep-wake cycle.
Rhythmicity	Regularity of sleep-wake cycle, feeding patterns, and elimination
Approach-withdrawal	Initial response to a new situation. (This may not be clear until two or three months.)
Adaptability	The ease with which the infant modifies and organizes responses in a new situation. (This may not be clear until two or three months.)
Intensity	The vigor of the child's responses to hunger, restraint, changing, and sensory stress.
Threshold	The level of sensory or social stimulation required to evoke a discernible response.
Mood	The balance of smiling and pleasurable interaction in contrast to fussing and irritation.
Distractibility	The ease with which the baby can be diverted from an activity by extraneous stimulation. (This may not be clear until two or three months.)
Attention span	The capacity to persist with an activity despite distraction or competing stimulation.

Results of the Study

Preliminary results have already been reported (Nurcombe, Howell, Rauh, et al., 1984; Nurcombe, Rauh, Howell, et al., 1984). Significant intervention effects were found, at six months, on measures of maternal role satisfaction, maternal self-confidence, and maternal perception of infant temperament, but not on measures of maternal attitudes to child-rearing or maternal psychopathology. No significant differences between the two LBW groups emerged at six and twelve months in Infant Mental Development as measured by the Bayley Scales.

An attempt was made to assess mother-infant interaction at four, six, and twelve months, using continuous microbehavioral event recording. No clear differentiation emerged, either among the three groups or within groups, and the measure was abandoned.

As to infant outcomes. a tantalizing near-significant trend appeared at 24 months on the Bayley Scales, and significant differences between the two LBW groups were evident at 36 and 48 months on the McCarthy Scales. The four-year findings, including intervention effects on cognitive development, will be fully described elsewhere (Rauh et al., forthcoming).

Conclusions

It is likely that the biological adversity associated with low birthweight obscures all other factors until the second year of life, when language and cognition begin to interweave and when psychomotor development recedes in importance as an index of developmental progress. The progressive emergence of language and information-processing after the second year is integral to the transactional explanation of our results. We contend that the MITP had an early beneficial effect on mother-infant interaction. Subsequently, progressively more favorable mother-infant transactions resulted in the boosting of maternal morale detected at six months. However, the biological insult associated with prematurity, and the inability of the nonverbal infant to demonstrate latent competence, initially obscured any effect of the MITP on infant development. An effect of the intervention could be seen only after the second year, when the infant had begun to exhibit both language and more complex cognitive abilities.

The implications of this study are intriguing. A more detailed analysis of results is required, together with a continued follow-up of the children, in order to determine whether the differences in outcome at 48 months have any significance for scholastic functioning. Furthermore, the apparently exceptional durability of the intervention effect, and the economy of the MITP in staff and time, indicate that it might have useful public health applications.

DISCUSSION

Peter Vietze: Barry, you seem to be ignoring the fact that you get differences between the two low-birthweight groups as early as twelve months. The differences may not be statistically significant, but there's a clear trend. This supports the view that change began in the first year and was not delayed until verbal consolidation had occurred.

Tiffany Field: Also, if you look at large samples of the low-SES infants in ICUs, without comparing interventions, you don't really begin to see a diminution of performance until around twelve months. It's as if the hard-wiring takes them through the first twelve months. SES doesn't begin to impact until after twelve months. So intervention may be compensating for SES.

Barry Nurcombe: We're not quite sure exactly what it was we did, but we did something with the mother (and through the mother with the baby) that allowed the mother to overcome the potentially adverse effects of low birthweight. In the long run, I suppose that one has to postulate that something happened to the wiring of that baby as a result of the intervention.

However, some results were counterintuitive. We expected a brilliant result at twelve months and a subsequent fading out. Instead we got the very reverse. I've worked in preschool intervention in Australia, and essentially what we got was early results and later washout—brilliant results gone within three years. That's what we expected from the Vermont study.

Robert Isaacson: Barry, you mentioned very early on that in dealing with intelligent mothers who had had premature children, you found that they seem to have an attitude that they had grown up being trained to *do* something, to be in control, and to accomplish something. Now, as mothers, they had to *be* something. Could you elaborate on that?

Barry Nurcombe: I'll elaborate by exaggerating it somewhat. Let's say a woman has spent all her life up to the age of thirty going to school, learning a professional job, and being successful. Now she's ready to have a baby. Everything in her life up to now has been part of a highly organized system. But suddenly, at 34 weeks, she delivers a premature baby. She has no clothes in the house (she was going to buy them at 37 weeks) and she feels out of control, whereas she usually has her life in tight control. She has to hang around the hospital, uncertain whether to go back to work, unsure whether she is going to lose the baby, and unclear whose fault it was that the baby was born so early. Then, with a week to go, somebody says, "Here's your baby." Now she has the sense that the buck stops with her. She hasn't had any of the preparation that occurs before a normal birth. But she's got the baby, and what she has to do with the baby is very different from what she did as a lawyer or a doctor. Essentially a mother has to *be* something. She has to *be* there, to *be* available. What she has to *be* isn't something you can teach, as at school. I have described the

Vermont program as though we instructed mothers like pupils, but what the intervention really did was to model caretaking and then pass it over to the mother, encouraging her to do what came naturally.

Arthur Parmelee: It has been my experience with our intervention program that if we set up a protocol like this, we can never follow it, because during those visits the mother wants to talk about something else, not about the things that we have in mind. Her attention may be focused on the fact that her husband isn't cooperating, they have to find a new apartment, and another child is ill. At that particular moment she is not prepared to talk about how she interacts with the baby. How did you cope with that?

Barry Nurcombe: Well, we played it by ear as we went along. We knew, of course, that the guidelines of the eleven-day intervention would often have to be modified in particular cases. There were some mothers who knew it all anyway and were involved because the toss of the coin had assigned them to the intervention group. But there were other mothers who took a long time to progress beyond the second day, because they were so preoccupied. Their minds were elsewhere, and they were jerky with the baby. Sometimes it was best to sit down with them and say, "Is there something on your mind?" and encourage them to talk about it.

Frances Horowitz: In your sample, you don't have highly stressed families. Many of the families were not—as families—disorganized in the care of the baby.

Barry Nurcombe: Some were quite significantly, but many were not.

Frances Horowitz: Then the positive effects of the intervention could carry on even after the intervention stopped, whereas in families that were highly disorganized for reasons other than having a premature baby, the effects would go away unless you continued the intervention. I don't know if that hypothesis makes sense.

Barry Nurcombe: It makes sense to me. We could look at that, actually, although I think the number of very stressed, disorganized women was relatively small. At six months we assessed the quality of support the mother received from her husband and family. We haven't yet looked at that predictively, but it may well interact with the intervention in an interesting way.

Arthur Parmelee: In all the families you selected the father was present, unlike many studies that deal with more impoverished mothers.

Berry Brazelton: But if you establish a relationship with the mothers, which you did in your program, then you have an intervention available for them at each return checkup.

Jennifer Buchwald: Barry, if you accept your data and say, yes, this intervention has indeed done something very dramatic that has persisted over three years, do you have an opinion about what aspect of the intervention might be most important?

Barry Nurcombe: I think that what Frances said yesterday is the essence of it: How can you help the baby frame the period of quiet alertness, and then make the best of it, meanwhile not overstressing the baby and remaining sensitive to the baby's varying availability during the interaction? That's the key. You've got to do a number of things to enable the period of quiet alertness to become better defined, and then you interact imaginatively. You play with the baby, and as time goes on in the first year more and more social interaction is possible. The quality of play, of mutual enjoyment, is the heart of the matter.

Edward Tronick: If you took your whole high-risk sample, interventions and controls, and looked at the extent to which the infants had resolved issues around state, some of your early interaction data might predict what mothers are still trying to do with their infants at four months. Some mothers may now be moving on to genuine interactive play, because their infants have resolved state regulation issues. Play and the like become important in your interventions, because you've already supported them in emerging tasks of development.

Barry Nurcombe: We put a lot of effort into our mother-infant evaluation, but it didn't pan out. Not to have a useful index of interaction was a terrible disappointment. It would have been elegant to have shown enhanced interaction following intervention, and subsequently improved development in mother and baby in a transactional spiral.

Cynthia Garcia Coll: But have you looked at the interaction data in terms of individual differences? In those dyads with better interactions, did the children perform better later? It might be that not every dyad was affected by the intervention.

Barry Nurcombe: We employed two approaches to assessing interaction. One was a global assessment scale (of which Peter Vietze was co-designer). The second involved microbehavioral observations. We could discriminate only the best six and the worst six dyads. The rest were a great mass in the middle. After sophisticated analyses of the data (which Barry Lester helped us with), nothing came of it.

Peter Vietze: Barry, you may be looking too early. To expect substantial interactional changes after your last contact with them may have been too hopeful. If you had gone to a year or even eighteen months, you might have found something different.

Barry Nurcombe: There are major behavioral sampling problems, also. At the time of the interactional analysis, a baby can be having a bad day. It is unclear whether the kind of twenty-minute recording that we did could possibly be representative.

EARLY INTERVENTION: WHAT DOES IT MEAN?*

T. Berry Brazelton, M.D.

I would like today to address some of the forces in development that can be harnessed to help the infant compensate for defects, either organic or behavioral, that might otherwise make him or her subject to failures in development. A mildly impaired infant may present disorganized behavior that makes him appear to be more impaired than he really is. I think the timing of intervention is critical, not only in addressing the strengths of assets with which the infant and the parents can overcome deficits but also, and maybe more critically, in reinforcing the positive self-image in that baby from the first, and in adding motivation toward recovery to optimal function. For example, by the time we identify a child with a learning disability at the age of four or five, the disability itself is no longer as much of a problem for the child's future as is his own image of himself and his built-up

*This paper is adapted from T.B. Brazelton, "Early Intervention: What Does It Mean?" in H.E. Fitzgerald, B.M. Lester, and M.W. Yogman (Eds.), *Theory and Research in Behavioral Pediatrics*, Vol. 1 (New York: Plenum Press, 1982). Used by permission.

expectation to fail. In our work at Children's Hospital, we can see this expectation to fail in children as young as eight months who come from nonreinforcing environments or who have basic problems of their own. It's built in very early, and it's dogging everything they do. So individuated programs oriented early to the particular baby are critical, because we must reinforce the baby's own sense of himself and how he's handling things.

Grieving interferes with a parent's ability to perceive and value the potential organization in a disordered baby. She grieves for the perfect baby she might have had and compares this baby to that. The programs that reach out to grieving or anxious parents must take into account the reasons for the defenses around their anxiety. An understanding of the forces for attachment and for grieving in caregivers is critical for an understanding of the normal forces for development in the infant. I do not believe it is as simple as some people say for a caregiver to get over the grief that is interfering with the kind of relationship that she can offer that child. In fact, it doesn't surprise me a bit that it takes nearly two years before you begin to get the sleeper effects that Nurcombe (1987, this volume) is demonstrating.

Assessing the Neonate

Much of my own thinking has come from work on the behavioral assessment of the neonate (Brazelton, 1973, 1984) and on the face-to-face work that I did with Tronick (Brazelton et al., 1975). The main thing that we've learned from those studies was that simple assessments are not enough. I also feel that using one assessment as a predictor is relatively worthless; we need at least two, probably three, for an accurate prediction.

The other thing we've learned from using the Neonatal Behavioral Assessment Scale (NBAS) is that if we allow parents to share it with us, they can begin to understand their impaired child and work for an environment that is appropriate to their child. We at Children's Hospital are now in the midst of a study of Intrauterine Growth Retarded (IUGR) babies. We are filming the parents as they watch us demonstrate the NBAS, and we then analyze which parts of the scale cause what we call "hitting the mark" and which ones don't. This will give us an idea of which parts of the scale are important to people, but I think we already know that it's the state changes and state maintenance that are the most critical to parents' understanding of their babies as well as to the handling of the babies.

We're seeing an interesting difference in the way the lower-SES (socioeconomic status) parents and the middle-class parents respond as they watch us demonstrate their babies. The lower-SES parents take longer to become involved. The middle-class parents are more receptive and watch intently from the first, and by the third time they are doing it with us. I think there is a significant difference in how we approach people across class and across individuals, and perhaps that should be part of our model.

An understanding of the forces that work toward a child's development is critical to understanding his failure and to any effort to prevent such failure. There are three sources of energy for developmental processes (see Figure 7). Of course the central nervous system's (CNS) maturation is the most powerful and the limiting one, but also the energizing one for future development.

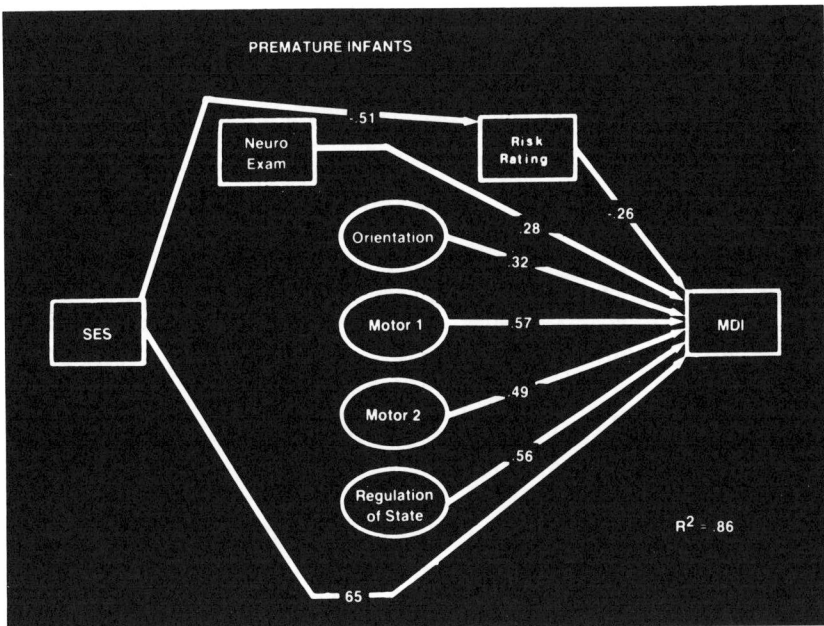

Figure 7. Three sources of energy for development

The next most important set of energies is the internal feedback system. These are the inborn programs of development that we are tapping into, now that we understand the neonate better. This internal programming, if you will, of both genetic endowment and intrauterine shaping provides goals and, then, a critical feedback system for the infant. As he works to achieve something, you can see it in his face when he reaches his goal. Even as a newborn, when he achieves success in quieting with use of his hand-to-mouth reflex his whole face lights up. To me this represents the closing of an internal feedback system that goes with the recognition of programs that are inborn.

The external feedback system is what we've been talking about at this Round Table, feedback from the environment. But it's when those two—the internal and the external—can lock that we are able to attain, first, a state of homeostasis and then a sense of achievement in the baby. The energy and drive are there in the baby to reach out for those feedback systems for himself. My own concept now is that learning how to regulate the internal feedback systems around his state of consciousness, and learning that he can control state for himself, may be the first real sense of achievement that a baby gets. We certainly see it in the baby and in the mother, when the mother and baby can lock together in a mutual rhythm of attention/withdrawal, attention/recovery. As they set up the approach/withdrawal rhythm necessary to prolonged attention, they both get a concept of how they are doing it. This kind of mastery within the dyad leads to a sense of competence in the baby.

Modes of Recovery

The opportunities for recovery from a CNS insult in immature brains are out of proportion to any of our earlier preconceptions about fixed CNS damage. But the immature nervous system has uncaptured pathways to take up impaired functions. If the environment can provide appropriate, nurturing information, the CNS will attempt to incorporate it and to learn from it. For the impaired infant, several modes of recovery function with these forces of development. Vicarious functioning, for instance, is one that intrigues me. We had a blind baby that we were following, and at eleven months the baby started lying in her crib rolling her head and going "Ah, ah, ah, ah, ah" in either direction. At this point we began to fear that she was autistic, because we were so sure she'd be brain-damaged, too. But instead, when at fourteen months she started walking, going "Ah, ah, ah, ah, ah," she never walked into furniture, and she walked through doors without touching the door jambs. This baby had started her sonar three months before she needed it. This use of auditory and kinesthetic mechanisms to replace her vision was an example of vicarious functioning. She was using other senses for a kind of vicarious functioning since she lacked vision.

Another mode of recovery is from the capture of the many redundant pathways available in the immature nervous system. I was taught in medical school that if you had a knocked-out pathway, that was it. Researchers now tell us that there are many redundant pathways in the immature nervous system that can replace impaired systems. If we pay attention to this concept and try to capture them by appropriate information to them in infancy, we can perhaps capture pathways that are intact and put them to use to substitute for the impaired ones.

What does appropriate mean in this context? What I mean is that if there is a damaged area in the brain, of course capillaries and neurons rush in to try to repair it. As they do, they set up a hypersensitive field around that area, which will then spread to the rest of the brain. All of us who have handled babies like this know that they are hypersensitive in most of their sensory and motor responses. But if we expect that and don't treat it as if it were abnormal but begin to gear our stimuli down to that kind of hypersensitivity, we can get the same responses that we do from a normal baby. Unless we can adapt our stimuli in a sensitive way to each baby's ability to handle them, we will overload these babies. We will fail to pay attention to the disorganization that could be captured for organization. Appropriate information to such a hypersensitive baby becomes quieter, less complex, and from one modality. Then the information can be utilized to assign pathways as yet uncaptured to the necessary function.

A Systems Approach

This leads me to a systems approach. We need to think of the different modalities in the baby as affecting each other in a sort of system. The baby is also embedded in the system of a family. All of these interact with each other. The importance of each modality in the baby interacting with each modality in the parent makes us need an interactional model to understand either the baby or the parent-infant system. We included in the interactional model the violation of the baby's expectation for his mother to react to him in a social play situation. We had seen how important was their expectation to interact. We saw what it meant to the baby to have the mother come in and fail to respond in the usual way. You could see the baby working very hard to restore the interaction, trying to recapture the mother. But you could also see what it meant to the mother; it was clearly painful to be violating this system. Thus, the intactness of the system as well as the cost of any violation within it becomes vital in understanding any failure in the baby or in the parent-infant system.

We have added a series of items to the NBAS, which we think now are probably critical toward looking at impaired or at-risk babies along with other items of the Scale (see Table 10). They are qualitative and represent what it costs a baby to pay attention, to react, to interact with his environment, and what it costs that baby to maintain state, to maintain autonomic control in order to react. We score the infant for robustness and endurance and also for how his effort is reflected in his motor tone when he has to give up. We also look at what it costs the examiner to get that baby into an interaction and maintain the baby's optimal interaction in the Neonatal Assessment. Examiners become indicators of the baby's future organization.

Table 10. NBAS Supplementary Items

Quality of alert responsiveness	Quality of alertness and attention responses
Cost of attention	Stress to motor, physiological, and state systems during elicitation of attention
Examiner persistence	Input supplied by the examiner to elicit behavioral responses
General irritability	Quality and range of irritability during the examination
Robustness and endurance	Fragility and energy level over the course of the examination
Regulatory capacity	Ability to respond to increasing levels of stimulation
State regulation	Ability to maintain levels of behavioral organization with increasing examination manipulations
Balance of motor tone	Variations in motor tone in upper and lower body
Reinforcement value of the infant's behavior	How appealing the infant was to the examiner

This in turn ought to suggest what it is going to cost the parent to assist the baby toward organization. And all of us who play with impaired babies know that the cost we are asking of parents is incredible. I believe it is critical to think about some of the things that parents have to go through when they have a disordered baby or a preemie. I equate their reaction to what Lindeman talked about in his seminal paper (1944) on the grief reaction. Lindeman said that adults who lose someone important automatically blame themselves, feel it was their fault, and try to repair it by saying "If I'd only done this, or if I'd only done that" in an effort to deal with their disappointment and grief. They take it personally and begin to feel depressed and withdrawn, defending themselves with three defenses: denial, projection, and detachment.

All these defenses distort a person's ability to look for and interact with the organizing developmental processes we are talking about. *Denial* is the most general and critical defense. For the mother, it distorts reality. When she is denying, she distorts the baby's behavioral cues and overreacts or underreacts. *Projection* can mean projecting onto everyone else "They know what to do but I don't," or the opposite—"I know what to do but you don't." Mothers put doctors and nurses up against the wall and get into locked battle with them. Finally, mothers detach from the baby, not because they don't care but because it hurts so much to care. I would expect those defenses to last a long time, not only because of the parents' own reparative needs but because of the violations of expected responses that they meet in a preterm or a disordered baby. The longer the parent/infant dyad is out of synchrony with each other, the longer it is going to take before they get out of the grief period and we begin to see recovery and sleeper effects.

The Touch Points

I run a teaching program at Harvard for pediatricians in which we are trying to understand the processes that parents must go through as they evolve as parents of a developing child, but also as caregivers. We've been looking at when it pays off for a pediatrician or nurse-practitioner to get into the parent/infant system, in a ten-minute intervention. We call these opportunities "touch points," points when the system would be open enough to let you in with appropriate information and allow you to make a difference to the future of that baby.

The first touch point we've been looking at is in the last trimester of the prenatal period. Sharing ten minutes with parents there amounts to about twelve hours of work that it might take to make a comparable relationship with these people later on. The second touch point is the perinatal period, where we use the Behavioral Assessment to demonstrate the baby to them as our mode of communication between parents and ourselves, because behavior is such a universal language. As soon as you begin to talk descriptively about what the baby is doing and what is going on underneath, the mother is locked onto you. We do not assess his behavior pejoratively, but descriptively.

Piaget (1952) pointed out to us that any developmental line goes in a burst of energy, followed by a leveling off and a consolidation, and then another burst. It appears to us that what leaves these systems open for intervention is that there is a disorganization just before there is a burst, and the disorganization in the baby or in the parent may make them available to us, to establish a relationship or pass on information. Maybe we ought to be looking for these disorganizing times to get into the system, not to teach but to join with the parents in their work, modeling and playing with behavior and talking in language they can understand.

The third touch point (all these follow biobehavioral shifts in the full-term baby) is at about three weeks, when the EEG shows some maturation and when colic is about to start as a part of the 24-hour rest-activity cycle. Right at that point, if you intervene you can prevent the anxiety in parents that colic creates. I can set up this same model for preventing sleeping or feeding disorders later on by using three or four such touch points in these areas in the first year. We need to think of our opportunities for entering the parent-infant system if we want to help parents. These are economical times for us, and it certainly might help us as professionals.

Predicting Outcomes

Barry Lester and I have been doing some work on an old study (Lester, Hoffman, & Brazelton, 1984) that has been very instructive. We had started working with these preterm babies when they got off supports. We demonstrated the NBAS to the parents at 36, 38, 40, 42, and 44 weeks' conceptional age. This was supposed to be a normative study, but it turned out to be an intervention study, because the parents never missed an observation. We could see how invested they were in modeling our behavior as we helped these babies to respond.

Our results at eighteen months have now been replicated at five years. SES, of course, is the biggest predictor to the Bayley Mental Development Index (MDI) at eighteen months. But we can add to the SES as a predictor by using the "recovery" drives of neonatal behavior as determined by repeated NBAS exams at 40, 42, and 44 weeks. The items that predicted were the baby's behavior—orientation, two aspects of motor behavior, and the use of state.

The risk rating for medical events with these high-risk infants—we used Parmelee's risk rating (Parmelee et al., 1975)—did predict if it was tied to SES. The neurological examination at 40 weeks—again Parmelee's examination—predicted at a low level. When all these factors are added to SES, we got a .85 prediction to MDI at eighteen months and .65 to the performance on the McCarthy scales at five years. There are predictions from the neonatal period. For the full-term or premature baby, the way the baby recovers from the stress of labor and delivery may well be the best predictor of future function. State is the best predictor from the neonatal assessment, and SES is the most important. What we have lacked, I think, is a systems approach to the kind of predictions we want to make. We need repeated assessments of the neonate as he recovers from labor and delivery. As he recovers, we can predict to this future organization. If we begin to pay attention to the interaction of all these, we may be talking about some genuinely predictive indicators for babies, both full-term and preterm.

DISCUSSION

Robert Isaacson: You talked about the supersensitivity spreading to the rest of the brain. I'd like to suggest that maybe it doesn't spread to all the rest of the brain but to certain of the systems that generally modulate the activities of the brain, and I think it would be very interesting if we could find some way of discovering which ones are involved. It seems to me that having a whole brain "supersensitive" doesn't make sense, but it does make sense to have some systems supersensitive and to have this correlate with behavioral anomalies. Maybe an undersensitive inhibitory system would be as tragic as a supersensitive system.

Berry Brazelton: Bob, speak a little bit to the two systems that seem to be locked—not only the intake of stimuli but the motor output. Often these hypersensitive babies are also hyperreactive in their motor and state controls as well.

Robert Isaacson: Yes, there is an animal model in which various forms of abnormal behaviors are found after the administration of opiate-like drugs to young animals. These drugs include morphine, codeine, and a codeine-like drug, an experimental codeione. The morphine produces a relatively long period of alert immobility, a "frozen state" of active attention to sights and sounds but an inhibition of movement. The codeione and codeine itself produce the opposite type of effective, enhanced motoric acts that are followed by a state of quiet sleep or rest. These effects can be observed when the drugs are given peripherally only until early adulthood. After that the codeine and codeine-like drugs seem to be ineffective. Behaviors that can be considered "restorative" or acting to decrease behavioral activation, in particular self-grooming, are found soon after the codeine and codeine-like drug are given, but only a long time after morphine, when the hyper-alert immobility dissipates. We believe grooming is a sure predictor that the animal is on the way to reestablishing neural homeostasis.

Berry Brazelton: There is a human model, you know—withdrawing babies of mothers who are hooked on the hard opiate substances and probably alcohol, too. They look like this as they withdraw.

Robert Isaacson: Well, one of the surprising things I've read in the literature is that some mothers who presumably were taking only codeine have babies who undergo apparent withdrawal. This is remarkable, since only 10 percent of codeine is demethylated to morphine. Therefore they must have been taking very high doses of codeine to produce a state of withdrawal in a newborn. Our evidence in animals is very clear that morphine and codeine act on quite different sets of receptors.

Barry Nurcombe: If a resourceful mother can do something effective with the baby that counteracts the ill effects of low birthweight and all that goes with it, it's got to have an ultimate neurological basis. Something must happen inside that baby's brain. Berry has alluded to some broad things, but I really can't conceive what actually must be happening. Can I tempt somebody to conjecture what it might be? I think it's time we started to conjecture about this. Is it purely a functional matter—that is, the baby's brain is perfectly okay but for reasons we don't fully understand the mother, or the environment, doesn't stimulate him, so he doesn't learn, and he turns out not so bright as he might be? Or is it in fact that there is structural abnormality and that a resourceful mother can circumvent it somehow or help the baby develop alternative pathways?

Anneliese Korner: Isn't the evidence accumulating that it's not so much the prematurity but the illnesses that follow the fact that the baby is premature that cause the damage—the respiratory distress and so on?

Barry Nurcombe: Whatever it is, something must affect the brain, structurally or functionally. I'm using low birthweight, but it's a catch-all for all the bad things that happen.

Robert Isaacson: I think that what has been ignored by us all is the extraordinarily potent effects of tropic factors, both neuronotropic and neuritotropic. NGF (neural growth factor) is one that most people know about, but there is some hot research on other types of brain stimulatory factors. Now, in the stress domain: if ACTH (adrenocorticotropin hormone) is being secreted by the organism as the trigger for stress, for every molecule of ACTH that's produced a molecule of Beta-endorphin is also produced, because they come from a common precursor and are split on a one-for-one basis. Consequently, stress induces a release of both ACTH and Beta-endorphin. Now that doesn't mean the effects of either of these two neuropeptides are the same, because the membrane effects which they produce last considerably longer than the persistence of their original chemical structures. The durations of the membrane effects of ACTH and Beta-endorphin are probably quite different from each other.

Infant animals given opiate receptor blocking drugs have brains considerably larger than those of control-treated animals. It would appear that we have largely ignored a very important regulator of brain size, namely the endogenous opiate system. I think we're living in a very exciting time. If we have a conference like this five years from now, we will know a great deal more about this.

Barry Lester: I think Barry's question is very important. As we have said, notions of brain plasticity are often used to justify early intervention, and in Berry's mention of the different mechanisms for recovery, certainly that's the implication. What Barry is asking is how that might work.

Barry Nurcombe: Is the trigger the perceptual experiences of, say, looking at the mother's face and being fixed and being engaged, or is it the affect that goes with it, or is it a mixture of certain sorts of percepts with strong affect that then releases tropic substances which cause dendritic growth, which then compensates for the damage?

Berry Brazelton: But why can't you postulate that when the baby gets himself organized, he senses it and realizes it? It seems to me that would be a far more powerful feedback system and learning precursor than getting it from the outside. I would think a lot of our intervention ought to be aimed at that indirect approach to the baby's systems, rather than putting in anything from the outside. In other words, I'd follow him, using his behavioral responses as our guide.

Barry Nurcombe: I guess I'm seeing the interaction as being the key. I'm sure babies can help to organize themselves, but I'm assuming that a high quality of direction helps the baby to do it quicker. But also it puts in something else we don't fully understand, and that's a complex perceptual and affective trigger to internal hormonal production, tropic substance, God knows what, but it seems to affect brain growth and maybe even compensatory brain growth.

Kathryn Barnard: Deirdre Blank has an interesting article about to come out in *Nursing Research*. She measured on the Spielberger State-Trait Anxiety Scale the mother's anxiety before and after feeding a newborn two days of age. She collected glucose and cortisol levels of the baby before and after the feeding. She found a relationship between the mother's anxiety and the baby's cortisol level after feeding. So there appears to be a process by which some of these affects do get communicated biochemically across people. Furthermore she proposes that infants of mothers with low pre-feeding anxiety have infants who both take in less milk and end the feeding with a higher post-feeding cortisol level, implying that these infants have their hunger needs met primarily by endogenous gluconeogenesis.

Robert Isaacson: I think corticosterone—or cortisol, depending on the species—is one of the major influences here. Landfield's evidence in aging is that corticosterone greatly reduces the dendritic branching and the spines of cells in the hippocampus. There is no reason to believe that this is unique to the aged animal. Another possibility, of course, is that high corticosterone levels are not as important as either the conditions that cause them to occur or their secondary effects on the release of hormones from the adrenal medulla. Furthermore, corticosterone or cortisol also changes the enzymatic coating of the intestines, such that the much larger proteins can enter, rather than just amino acids. The final step in degradation of proteins is on these surfaces. When you have high stress conditions there may in fact be subtle changes in nutrition as well.

Michael Schwartz: Actually, the corticosterone story is a little difficult, though, because there is a body of literature from some ten or twelve years ago demonstrating that in immature rats administration of corticosterone actually increases dendritic growth and spine growth.

Craig Ramey: I was going to answer Barry's question in a more concrete way, because we may have a tantalizing opportunity to do something to get an answer. In our longitudinal intervention research, which I will be describing a little later, we have shown that we can produce differences in outcomes with children. One way we have gone is to draw blood, beginning with cord blood and then blood every three months, and store it frozen. We collected enough so that we then set some aside. Is there anything you can think of that could be assayed through blood that might serve as a marker for brain changes?

Robert Isaacson: Well, you've said the magic word. There are several things, depending on how much blood you've got. Certainly alpha-fetoprotein is one that I think ought to be assayed as an index of the brain's development. It's a protein that is essentially absent in the adult brain. If the adult has cancer, alpha-fetoprotein may appear in measurable amounts. But it's always present in the fetal period, and then it declines rather rapidly after birth. It could be a very interesting index of how brain development is progressing. There are some other proteins, particularly growth factors, that could be used as indices of brain growth. We now have radioimmunoassays for most of them. I think it would be very exciting to look at their relation to brain development.

EARLY INTERVENTION: WHY, FOR WHOM, HOW, AT WHAT COST?

Craig T. Ramey, Ph.D.,
Donna M. Bryant, Ph.D.,
and Tanya M. Suarez, Ph.D.

When the concept of intervention is applied to human development, the goal is usually to enhance functioning or to prevent some unwanted condition. During the past twenty years, the United States has committed itself to early intervention for young children who are socioeconomically, educationally, or physically disadvantaged. Federal legislation such as the Economic Opportunity Act of 1964, which contained Head Start, and the Education of the Handicapped Act of 1975, which included the Handicapped Children's Early Education Program, provided for a variety of developmentally supportive services, with early education at the core of the effort. A great deal of scientific knowledge and practical experience has accumulated since these legislative commitments were made. The purpose of this paper is to summarize what has been learned about early educational intervention and to recommend future public policy and associated research.

Why Intervene Early?

The idea that early experience affects later development is an old one, yet the importance of early experience has been advanced only intermittently in the history of Western thought. More frequently, concepts other than early experience have been regarded as central to development.

In the nineteenth century, predeterminism was advanced by Galton and other proponents of the primacy of heredity in development. Predeterminism acknowledged maturational changes but held that these changes were relatively encapsulated and consequently unaffected by early experience (Gottlieb, 1971a).

In the 1950s the early experience paradigm became the chief competitor of the predeterministic view of development. Evidence from three major streams of investigation flowed together to establish the premise of the primacy of early experience: (1) Freud's theory of psychosexual development; (2) ethological concepts and especially the phenomenon of imprinting (Lorenz, 1937), which were interpreted as representing a unique predisposition for learning, present for only a brief critical period; and (3) Hebb's (1949) neuropsychological theory for the existence of critical periods in intellectual as well as social development. Subsequent investigations with animals revealed that variations in early experiences affected both the organization and the biological bases of behavior (Thompson & Heron, 1954; Krech, Rosenzweig, & Bennett, 1960).

As the early experience paradigm took hold, the conceptualization of the impact of early experience was broadened and deepened. Initially, early experience was seen to predispose an individual toward a certain personality structure and predictable ways of responding. Later, with the concept of critical periods, early experience was seen to impart stable and irreversible neurological consequences that could set a ceiling for later problem-solving behavior (see, for example, Harlow, 1958). Although the empirical support for this notion was scant and limited to investigations with laboratory animals, this interpretation of the effects of early experience formed the theoretical basis for much of the work done in the area of human intellectual development in the past two decades.

The implications of critical-period research were assimilated in the influential educational theories of J. McVicker Hunt and Benjamin Bloom. Hunt's concept of the match (1961) was an application of Piaget's stage model of intellectual development and assigned a greater role to the characteristics of the environment than to the hereditary make-up of the individual. Hunt saw developmental advances as the result of the child's successful interaction with increasingly complex stimuli. In his view, then, adequate intellectual development depended upon the child's receiving specific stimulation at appropriate points in development. Although Hunt's general thesis did not postulate critical periods, it implied that early experiences were particularly important.

Bloom (1964) made two points that focused on preschool intervention as a critical period. First, he argued that intellectual growth occurred most rapidly in the first three years of life and tapered off by the time the child entered grade school. Second, he specifically argued that the first five years of life were a critical period for intellectual development. Only during the early years of life, in his opinion, was intellectual development characterized by plasticity. Consequently, these years provided the major and perhaps the only opportunity to facilitate development by enriching the child's environment.

According to the early experience paradigm, intellectual deficiencies arose from the inadequacies in the child's environment, deficiencies that could be eradicated by providing enrichment programs during the preschool years. Yet as programs designed to provide this education were developed and tried in the 1960s, early education was judged not to have kept its central promise. A nationwide evaluation of Project Head Start concluded that no permanent benefits with regard to intelligence could be found. The initial positive effects of Head Start attendance were judged to be moderate (Cicirelli, 1969). A similar pattern of results was discerned from an influential secondary analysis of the results of other early intervention programs (Bronfenbrenner, 1975).

The resulting attack on enrichment programs indirectly became a battle concerning the early experience paradigm. Jensen (1969) attributed depressed intellectual development in socially disadvantaged and black children to genetic inferiority rather than environmental defects—a retreat to a predeterministic point of view—and considered early educational intervention doomed to ineffectiveness.

More recently, however, development has been conceptualized as a continuous process, a cumulative series of transactions between individuals and their environments (see, for example, Ramey, Trohanis, & Hostler, 1982). This view of development still sees the early years of human life as highly significant for later development, for two main reasons. First, home environments tend to remain stable over time in the absence of systematic intervention (Gottfried, 1984). Second, potential plasticity in later development is less likely to be capitalized on, since society tends to associate learning experiences such as schooling with the earlier years. Certain developmental tasks are therefore less likely to be accomplished after a specific age, even if it is theoretically possible.

Several recent experimental findings buttress our case for a cumulative-transactional model of development. First, individual differences in home environments have been shown to be stable during the preschool years not only in disadvantaged homes (Yeates et al., 1983) but in advantaged homes (Gottfried, 1984) and in socioeconomically mixed samples (Elardo, Bradley, & Caldwell, 1977). Thus, stable individual differences in home environments are not merely artifacts of a family's socioeconomic status.

Second, in the absence of intervention, individual differences in home environments are additive over the preschool years in accounting for increasing percentages in variation in IQ scores until age four, whereas maternal IQ accounts for a relatively constant percentage of variation in IQ scores (Ramey, Yeates, & Short, 1984). Thus, environments appear to be cumulative in their influence on intellectual development.

Third, children's characteristics contribute to the creation of the home environments that they occupy (Zeskind & Ramey, 1978, 1981; Breitmayer & Ramey, 1984).

For Whom Should We Intervene?

There are at least three types of young children likely to need access to special early intervention: (1) children at risk for developmental retardation because of medical conditions such as genetic damage or low birthweight; (2) children at risk for developmental retardation because of poor home environments; and (3) children at risk because of parental abuse or neglect.

It has been hypothesized for some time that children with biological damage detectable at birth have a spectrum of developmental outcomes that can be influenced by the quality of the environment to which those children are exposed (Sameroff & Chandler, 1975). It is also known that if children who are biologically healthy at birth are exposed to inadequate or inappropriate stimulation, they will begin to evidence developmental delays during the preschool period (Ramey, MacPhee, & Yeates, 1982). This delay is found almost exclusively among economically and educationally disadvantaged families. It is also more frequently found among blacks than whites (Finkelstein & Ramey, 1980). Thus, there is clearly inequality in the incidence and prevalence of retarded development. We have information that will help us select children most in need of early intervention (Ramey & MacPhee, in press), but we must continue to monitor young children at risk and to conduct further research in order to be better able to identify the children who would benefit from early educational intervention.

How To Intervene

One of the best-kept secrets in psychology and education is that early intervention works! Recent reviews of the early intervention literature have revealed at least nineteen studies in which children were randomly assigned to educationally treated or control groups (Ramey et al., 1982; Ramey, Bryant, & Suarez, in press; Bryant & Ramey, 1984). From the evidence in these projects, one can conclude that: (1) early intervention can reduce grade retention and special class placement during public school, and that while it has not resulted in permanent changes in IQ, significant elevations exist, typically for several years after early intervention is terminated (Darlington et al., 1981); (2) more educationally intense programs produce larger and longer-lasting developmental changes than less intense programs (Ramey & Bryant, 1982); and (3) structured intervention programs lead to better cognitive outcomes than unstructured programs (Karnes, 1975).

These conclusions provide clues about how to intervene. The developing child and the child's family are elements of a larger developmental system that includes the household, the neighborhood, and society. The experiences that the child has in the presence of adult caregivers provide him with what Feuerstein (1977) has called mediating learning experiences, which form the young child's primary knowledge acquisition device. Early childhood educators concerned with enhancing the development of high-risk children have focused on either the child, the parent, or the parent-child relationship as the target for developmental change. Programs, conducted either within children's own homes or within educational or developmental centers, have varied considerably in the extent to which they treated the family as a system embedded within a larger network.

Four major approaches can be distinguished, on a continuum of educational practice:

1. *Critical event or critical attribute approach.* These programs focus either upon providing services during a specific critical period or upon encouraging the development of a specific attribute that will allegedly influence other attributes positively and ultimately result in normal development.

2. *Enrichment technique.* These programs are designed to provide an exposure to developmentally enhancing experiences considered to be lacking in the home environment.

3. *Compensatory education.* These programs are designed to reach the same goals as regular education but using alternative pathways, such as the use of a communication board to teach language to a child with a severe speech impairment.

4. *Systems-integrative approach.* This approach recognizes the multiple forces, including genetic, psychological, sociological, and economic, that affect the child's development and creates interventions timed and placed to have multiple and synergistic effects on the child and on the child's environment.

The Costs of Intervention

Effective early interventions are expensive. There is no quick cure for delayed development. Early intervention is a field that has existed for only the past twenty years, and the pioneers in this field are largely self-taught. There is a need both to celebrate the accomplishments that have been made so far and to find systematic avenues to recruit sophisticated new professionals. We should not assume that the knowledge is on hand with which to educate effective psychologists, teachers, social workers, or pediatricians. We are also badly in need of technical assistance activities that will provide in-service training to existing early interventionists. At the same time, our colleges of education, psychology, social work, and medicine need to produce the next generation of people who will be able to see more clearly what needs to be done in research and clinical service and to act in an even more comprehensive and coordinated fashion.

While we are in the process of developing cost-effective models of early intervention, there is a major cost-saving step that we take: to make better use of early intervention sites as multipurpose family centers in which to integrate the delivery of health, education, and social services to families.

Conclusions

We recommend five guidelines concerning the operation of early intervention programs:

1. Practitioners should assume that detrimental conditions will not change. High-risk children should be placed in systematic educational programs as soon as the risk status is verified.

2. Special emphasis should be placed on risk indicators in the child's natural ecology, not solely on the child's cognitive or social performance.

3. High-risk children should remain in systematic educational programs at least until there is evidence of a positive change in risk indicators.

4. Educators should try to involve parents meaningfully in the child's educational program.

5. Systematic variations in educational curricula, format, and timing should be tried, with the aim of increasing program effectiveness and client satisfaction.

Whichever intervention approach is adopted, there are at least four major criteria by which programs should be evaluated. First, are they enjoyable? Well-intentioned but grim programs will not attract and hold those who are most needy. Second, are they flexible? If they do not take into account the needs of individual families, they are not likely to be effective. Third, are they comprehensive? If an agency seeks to serve a diverse clientele with a mixture of biological and environmental handicaps, it must draw on the knowledge of nutritionists, health professionals, social workers, psychologists, occupational therapists, and physical therapists. Finally, are the programs effective in positively modifying the development of children and families? Well-intentioned but ineffective programs do not deserve public support.

We as scientists must be available to help inform debates about public policy alternatives. We should also realize that the formulation of public policy and good science almost always proceed by fundamentally different rules. We must take every opportunity to understand the policy concerns and constraints of elected officials and to inform them of what science can and cannot legitimately do. There is, however, no inherent contradiction between excellent science and excellent participation in the policy arena.

DISCUSSION

Barry Nurcombe: Craig, is it not fair to say that most of the time the early advances that are school-based fizzle out if you don't involve the families? that if there isn't a change in the family system paralleling changes in the child, you get counteracting effects by elementary school?

Craig Ramey: That's a very frequently made statement, but it's unsupported by the literature. I believe we certainly should support families, but I've torn all the studies apart, down to the level of getting almost raw data from everybody, and I can't do an analysis showing that that idea is borne out by existing data.

Barry Nurcombe: But isn't it true that the effects of these programs tend to wash out?

Craig Ramey: There are some washout effects in that IQ scores come together, but Lazar and Darlington, of the Consortium for Longitudinal Studies, have shown that there are substantial lasting effects on reduction in grade retention and special class placement.

Frances Horowitz: That monograph also shows various kinds of empowerment of the parents. Many of these programs did not focus upon the family, but somehow the child's competence helped to empower the parents, particularly in terms of their subsequent involvement in the schools.

Peter Vietze: There are studies in the literature that do have washout effects. In fact, in the Early Childhood Consortium, most of the IQ effects seem to wash out by grade 3 or 4. But those were all preschool interventions that started at about the age of four and were trying to reverse whatever happened in the first four years. Karl White has done an evaluation of all the early intervention studies, and he did not find a parent component to be a crucial ingredient. And he looked at a great many different variables. He's now trying to do sixteen randomized clinical trials around the country with different kinds of children at different ages with different mixes of parent involvement. It's an exciting prospect, because it's really the first time anybody has attempted to titrate different variables. Ira Gordon tried to do that, systematically varying parent involvement, age of beginning, and kind of program, and unfortunately he died before he was able to finish that work.

Craig Ramey: In the Abecedarian Project, which began at entry to kindergarten, we randomly split the preschool groups. One-half gets an intervention over the first three years at public school and one-half has what the public school ordinarily offers. So we are soon going to be able to address the early versus later intervention issue.

Frances Horowitz: In 1973 Lucy Peyton and I reviewed all the Head Start and various other intervention programs to that date, and we came to exactly the same conclusion as Craig—that the effects were in proportion to the intensity of the program. Many of these were rather poor programs—quickly mounted and poorly designed—and in many of these quick and dirty intervention programs that occurred in the late 1960s, the effects did wash out in terms of school achievement by second or third grade. It is both the intensity and, I'm convinced, the quality of the educational program and the thoughtfulness behind the curriculum that matter. If you do this, you have to do it seriously. How much you directly involve the parents or indirectly affect them may not be the critical variable, but rather the quality of the educational program, especially when you're dealing with children who do not appear to be biologically insulted. One of the differences between the preterm, high-risk infants that most of us have talked about and the kind of population Craig is talking about is that the interventions are coming at different developmental points with different organismic needs. Much of our worry about things like state may be more critical for the more biologically fragile organisms, while the intense educational programs are the things that are going to make the difference for children who come from disadvantaged, socioeconomically poor families.

Craig Ramey: One of the conditions that we studied in one of our early intervention projects—Project CARE—was a comparison between a day care-based approach with the same curriculum delivered through a home visit format and with appropriate control families. All those children are now in public school. We have absolutely no evidence on any variable that we've ever measured that we've changed the attitudes, beliefs, or behavioral styles of the parents, and the performance of the children in the Home Visit Group falls uncannily on top of the scores of the control group. There is absolutely no positive developmental effect that we have been able to detect associated with participation in the Home Visit program. Please understand that I'm restricting my generalization only to very disadvantaged families with children who were biologically intact at birth. You might get a totally different kind of response for low-birthweight children or children who are handicapped in other ways.

I think there's a public policy implication. There is now a very strong belief in this country that intervention programs should work through parents. I share that belief. But if by doing that you don't accomplish the goal of preventing the child from falling down developmentally, you'd better add something to that. I think we're holding onto a romantic notion that we can support the family through a kind of verbal mechanism. We have to do more than that.

Kathryn Barnard: I've been working with a parallel type of population. We have been trying to work through the family and strengthen the social competencies of the mother, and it is now my feeling that that is not enough. We find that although the mothers can change, it takes a long time. By the time the mothers are better in terms of interaction and stimulation, it's too late for the baby. So I would agree that with very deprived, poorly educated mothers, it is somewhat unrealistic to expect family enrichment programs, parental support, or parent education to do the job that needs to be done of improving the environment and the conditions for supporting development of the child.

Craig Ramey: I keep waiting for some good evidence that parent-oriented, parent-mediated programs produce a big effect. Unfortunately, the only evidence that exists comes from tragically flawed studies, and the better the study, the smaller the difference.

Kathryn Barnard: I do think, though, that maybe one of the things we need to think about is a combination of education for the child and work with the families.

Craig Ramey: Well, I thought that, too. One of the conditions in Project CARE took the same child development center program that existed for the Abecedarian project and added to it a home visit component. The same home visit component was delivered by itself to another group. There is no difference between the child development center plus home visit group and the child development center group by itself.

Kathryn Barnard: But maybe the home-centered program shouldn't focus on the child's education. The home program should focus on building the competency of the parents.

Craig Ramey: It did. It had a dual focus. It was not just a program to go in and do the same thing with the child; it was both to help the families deal with some of their life problems as adults and in addition to teach them some specific things that they could do to help their child.

Tiffany Field: We too found in our comparisons that home-based programs didn't work very well. It wasn't until we actually paid the mothers a salary that we got the mothers to move off dead center. I just think it's unrealistic to think that you can really do anything to change the socioeconomic status of these mothers unless you give them jobs.

APPENDIX: GUIDELINES FOR STIMULATION OF PRETERM INFANTS

Before the early 1960s, the preterm infant was viewed as too fragile to handle stimulation. Caregivers were therefore told to handle the infant as little as possible. A reexamination of the literature on the effects of maternal deprivation, however, raised concerns that the preterm infant was deprived of stimulation, in an incubator seen as a sensory isolation chamber. This thinking led to a "more is better" approach to help the infant overcome the supposed potential deficits in information processing.

More recently it has been recognized that the nursery environment provides not only light and sound stimulation but patterned visual and auditory stimulation as well. Today, because of high technology and aggressive medical care, particularly that used with very small preterm infants, there is a concern that overstimulation may be a problem, and minimal handling is increasingly being recommended. The question is no longer whether stimulation for preterm infants is indicated. The preterm is stimulated. The questions are, stimulation for whom? what type? how much? how often? for what purpose? at what (post-conceptional/developmental) age?

It is also important to describe the population with whom these Guidelines are intended to be used: preterm infants in special care nurseries from initial admission to hospital discharge. This is a heterogeneous population that includes very low birthweight ($<$1,500 grams or $<$1,000 grams) infants, as well as those up to 2,500 grams. The smaller infants are more likely to be sick and to require the most medical intervention. The kinds of illnesses they experience also describe many subgroups of preterm infants, such as those with CNS insults (intraventricular hemorrhage, hydrocephalus) and those with respiratory problems (hyaline membrane disease, bronchopulmonary dysplasia). The small-for-gestational-age preterm is another subgroup. Note that we do not label all these groups as "at risk." Such a term is too general. Nonetheless the stimulation given to these infants must be carefully considered.

The Johnson & Johnson Pediatric Round Table Guidelines are an attempt to provide recommendations, based on our current state of knowledge, regarding stimulation of the hospitalized preterm infant. While they may have implications for the preterm infant after discharge from hospital, they were not developed for that purpose. They are not meant as a set of final statements; these recommendations will change as our knowledge base changes. And we recognize that these Guidelines make further demands on an already difficult situation. But they are offered in terms of our goal to provide the best possible care to these infants.

The following Guidelines were developed as a result of broad multidisciplinary discussion by all participants in the Round Table on Infant Stimulation:

1. Intervention studies with preterm infants have come from a variety of theoretical as well as atheoretical approaches, sometimes with conflicting results. It cannot be overemphasized that neither short-term nor long-term effects have been adequately demonstrated and that the mechanisms by which the techniques are thought to work are often not understood. There is a strong need for interdisciplinary research to define more accurately specific subgroups of preterm infants and to understand their course of development, the processes of their behavioral development, the physical, physiological, and neurophysiological basis of their development, the effects of the social and physical ecology of the special care nursery on development, and the mechanisms by which stimulation affects short-term and long-term development.

2. There is a strong interdependence between physiological and developmental processes that is critical for the care of the preterm infant and must be understood to determine appropriate intervention strategies. Research to study normal as well as abnormal human brain development in infants is

critical. In addition we need a better understanding of developmental changes in the brain as the infant approaches term gestational age, the effects of stimulation on the developing brain, and the relationships between the brain and behavior.

3. Advances in animal research have led to popular notions about the plasticity of the brain that have been used to inform intervention with preterm infants. However, "brain plasticity" is not a simple or unitary concept. In some areas, changes at a given structural-functional level can be produced by external stimulation; in other areas development may proceed independent of external stimulation. It would not be appropriate to base specific or direct intervention strategies on this work at this time.

4. Preterm infants are differentially sensitive to stimulation depending on their conceptional age, illness, and individual makeup. The physiologic homeostasis and immature brain of the preterm infant may be more vulnerable to excessive, inappropriate, or mistimed stimulation. Since we do not know how to relate the type of stimulation to the infant's level of brain development, the very immature infant probably should be protected from stimulation that could destabilize physiological homeostasis.

5. As the healthy preterm infant becomes less fragile and approaches term, the issue of what is appropriate stimulation can be considered. Stimulation should be related to the developmental level and the needs of the individual infant and to the specific purpose for which the intervention is intended.

6. Infant behavioral cues can be used to determine appropriate interventions for the individual infant. Signs of stress or avoidance behaviors indicate that stimulation should be terminated. Positive behaviors indicate that stimulation is appropriate.

7. Stimulation is not a unitary concept, and when it is used, the various parameters of stimulation need to be considered. These include the amount, type, timing, patterning, and quality of the stimulation. In addition, the choice of modalities and the number of modalities stimulated are important. Multimodal stimulation may be more stressful to the infant than stimulation in a single modality.

8. Stimulation may have both short-term and long-term effects on development, both of which need to be studied. Short-term effects may include changes in the infant's clinical course, physiological functioning, sleep-wake behavior, and interactive behavior. It is recommended that physiological monitoring that could indicate signs of stress (heart rate, respiration, pCO_2) accompany stimulation. Long-term outcome should be evaluated with measures of personality, affect, and temperament in addition to traditional measures such as morbidity, physical growth, and mental and cognitive function.

9. From a developmental perspective, once physiological homeostasis is stabilized, the organization of state is the next critical step as the healthy preterm approaches term. State organization includes both sleep states and awake states (alertness and crying), which are thought to be fundamentally different. State organization implies the ability to remain in a well-defined state for significant periods of time and the smoothness of transition from one state to the next. Effective interventions should be aimed at facilitating the infant's control of state organization.

10. The next developmental step following the control of state organization is the infant's ability to engage the social and inanimate environment. This step may not occur until after the infant reaches term. The stimulation that is provided should support information-processing abilities. At the same time it should be recognized that earlier accomplishments may still be fragile. As intervention strategies are implemented, attention should be paid to possible vulnerabilities in the infant, as indicated by changes in state, motor, and posturing behavior. These behavioral cues should be taught to caregivers and parents to aid their implementation of these strategies without stressing the infant.

11. Intervention with the preterm infant should be organized in the form of an individualized developmental plan to parallel the pediatric plan. The developmental plan should be constructed as a psychosocial intervention to include the parents and other immediate family members and to acknowledge the socioeconomic, cultural, and home environmental factors that will determine the family context in which the infant will be reared. The developmental plan

should include assessment of the infant's behavior, working with parents around the infant's medical and behavioral status, and helping the parents to deal with their own feelings, as well as discharge planning and follow-up. The developmental plan should involve an interdisciplinary team that includes input from medicine, nursing, psychology, physical and occupational therapy, child life, and social work.

12. There is a need for interdisciplinary training programs in psychosocial intervention with preterm infants. These programs should emphasize developmental processes, the interplay between developmental and physiological processes, and the role of the caregiving environment. Such training cannot be accomplished by packaged stimulation courses that last for only a few days. It requires extensive didactic and practical cross-disciplinary training. Perhaps a new discipline is needed.

REFERENCES

Ahmann, P.A., Lazzara, A., Dykes, F.D., Brann, A.W., & Schwartz, J.F. 1980. Intraventricular hemorrhage in the high-risk preterm infant: Incidence and outcome. *Annals of Neurology* 7(2):118-124.

Akiyama, Y., Schulte, F.J., Schultz, M.A., & Parmelee, A.H., Jr. 1969. Acoustically evoked responses in premature and full term newborn infants. *Electroencephalography and Clinical Neurophysiology* 26:371-380.

Als, H., Lester, B.M., Tronick, E.Z., & Brazelton, T.B. 1982. Manual for the assessment of the preterm infant's behavior. In H.E. Fitzgerald, B.M. Lester, & M.W. Yogman (Eds.), *Theory and research in behavioral pediatrics* (Vol. 1). New York: Plenum Press.

Als, H., Tronick, E., & Brazelton, T.B. 1978. Manual for the assessment of preterm and high risk infants: An extension of the Brazelton Scale. Unpublished manuscript, Children's Hospital Medical Center, Boston.

Altemeier, W.A., Vietze, P.M., Sherrod, K.B., Sandler, H.M., Falsey, S., & O'Connor, S. 1979. Prediction of child maltreatment during pregnancy. *Journal of the American Academy of Child Psychiatry* 18:205-218.

Amiel-Tison, C. 1968. Neurological evaluation of the maturity of newborn infants. *Archives of Disease in Childhood* 43:89-93.

Anderson, B.J., & Vietze, P.M. 1977. Early dialogues: The structure of reciprocal infant-mother vocalization. In S. Cohen & T.J. Comiskey (Eds.), *Child development: A study of growth processes.* 2d ed. Itasca, Ill.: Peacock.

Anderson, B.J., Vietze, P.M., Faulstich, G., & Ashe, M.L. 1978. Observation manual for assessment of behavior sequences between infant and mother: Newborn to 24 months. *JSAS Catalog of Selected Documents in Psychology* 8:31 (Ms. no. 1672).

Bakeman, R., & Brown, J.V. 1977. Behavioral dialogues: An approach to the assessment of mother-infant interaction. *Child Development* 48:195-203.

Barbas, H., & Mesulam, M-M. 1981. Organization of afferent input to subdivisions of area 8 in the rhesus monkey. *Journal of Comparative Neurology* 200:407-431.

Barnard, K.E. 1973. The effects of stimulation on the sleep behavior of the premature infant. In M. Batey (Ed.), *Western Journal for Communicating Nursing Research* (Vol. 6). Boulder, Col.: WICHE.

Barnard, K.E. 1980. Sleep organization and motor development in prematures. In E.J. Sell (Ed.), *Follow-up of the high risk newborn: A practical approach.* Springfield, Ill.: Charles C. Thomas.

Barnard, K.E., & Bee, H.L. 1983. The impact of temporally patterned stimulation on the development of preterm infants.*Child Development* 54:1156-1167.

Barnard, K.E., Hammond, M.A., Sumner, G.A., Kang, R., Johnson-Crowley, N., Snyder, C., Spietz, A., Blackburn, S., Brandt, P., & Magyary, D. 1987. Helping parents with preterm infants: Field test of a protocol. *Early Child Development and Care* 27:255-290.

Bates, J.E., Freeland, C.A., & Lounsbury, M.L. 1979. Measurement of infant difficultness. *Child Development* 50:794-803.

Beardslee, C.I. 1976. The sleep-wakefulness pattern of young hospitalized children during naptime. *Maternal-Child Nursing Journal* 5:15-24.

Bench, J., & Parker, A. 1971. Hyper-responsivity to sounds in the short-gestation baby. *Developmental Medicine and Child Neurology* 13:15-19.

Berg, W.K., & Berg, K.M. 1987. Psychophysiological development in infancy: State, startle, and attention. In J.D Osofsky (Ed.), *Handbook of infant development.* New York: Wiley.

Birnholz, J.C., & Benacerraf, B.R. 1983. The development of human fetal hearing. *Science* 222:516-518.

Blackburn, S. 1978. Sleep and awake states of the newborn. In *Early parent-infant relationships.* New York: National Foundation—March of Dimes.

Blackburn, S., & Barnard, K.E. 1985. Analysis of caregiving events in preterm infants in the special care unit. In A. Gottfried & J. Gaiter (Eds.), *Infant stress under intensive care.* Baltimore: University Park Press.

Bloom, R. 1964. *Stability and change in human characteristics.* New York: Wiley.

Bourgeois, J-P., Goldman-Rakic, P.S., & Rakic, P. 1985. Synaptogenesis of prefrontal cortex: Quantitative EM analysis in pre- and postnatal rhesus monkeys. *Society for Neuroscience Abstracts* 11:501.

Brazelton, T.B. 1962. Observations of the neonate. *Journal of the American Academy of Child Psychiatry* 1(1):38-58.

Brazelton, T.B. 1973. *Neonatal Behavioral Assessment Scale. Clinics in Developmental Medicine* no. 50. Philadelphia: Lippincott.

Brazelton, T.B. 1975. Newborn behavior. In E. Philips, J. Barnes, & M. Newton (Eds.), *Scientific foundations of obstetrics and gynecology.* London: William Heinemann.

Brazelton, T.B. 1978. Introduction. In A.J. Sameroff (Ed.), Organization and stability of newborn behavior: A commentary on the Brazelton Neonatal Behavior Assessment Scale. *Monographs of the Society for Research in Child Development* 43(5-6), serial no. 177.

Brazelton, T.B. 1984. *Neonatal Behavioral Assessment Scale.* 2d ed. Philadelphia: Lippincott.

Brazelton, T.B., Tronick, E.Z., Adamson, L., Als, H., & Wise, S. 1975. Early mother-infant reciprocity. *Ciba Foundation Symposium,* no. 33. Amsterdam: Elsevier.

Breitmayer, B., & Ramey, C.T. 1984. Biological nonoptimality and quality of postnatal environment as codeterminants of intellectual development. *Child Development* 57:1151-1165.

Bronfenbrenner, U. 1975. Is early intervention effective? In M. Guttentag & E.L. Struening (Eds.), *Handbook of evaluation research* (Vol. 2). Beverly Hills, Calif.: Sage Publications.

Brown, G.M., & Martin, J.B. 1974. Corticosterone, prolactin, and growth hormone responses to handling and new environment in the rat. *Psychosomatic Medicine* 36(3):241-247.

Brown, J.V., & Bakeman, R. 1979. Relationships of human mothers with their infants during the first year of life: Effects of prematurity. In R.W. Bell & W.P. Smotherman (Eds.), *Maternal influences on early behavior.* Holliswood, N.Y.: Spectrum.

Brown, M.C., Jansen, J.K.S., & Van Essen, D. 1976. Polyneural innervation of skeletal muscle in newborn rats and its elimination during maturation. *Journal of Physiology* 261:387-422.

Bryant, D.M., & Ramey, C.T. 1984. Prevention-oriented infant education programs. *Journal of Children in Contemporary Society* 7(1):17-35.

Buchwald, J.S. Generators. 1982. In E.J. Moore (Ed.), *Bases of auditory brainstem evoked responses.* New York: Grune & Stratton.

Buchwald, J.S. Animal models of event-related potentials. In press. In J. Rohrbaugh, R. Parasuraman, & R. Johnson (Eds.), *Event-related potentials of the brain.*

Buchwald, J.S., & Shipley, C. In press. Development of auditory evoked potentials in the kitten. In R.N. Aslin (Ed.), *Advances in neural and behavioral development* (Vol. 2). Norwald, N.J.: Ablex.

Cicirelli, V. 1969. *The impact of Head Start: An evaluation of the effects of Head Start on children's cognitive and affective development.* Athens, Ohio: Westinghouse Learning Corp.

Colombo, J. 1986. *Toward a characteristic view of the newborn and young infant.* Unpublished paper. The University of Kansas.

Cornell, E.H., & Gottfried, A.W. 1976. Intervention with premature human infants. *Child Development* 47:32-39.

Courchesne, E. 1979. From infancy to adulthood: The neurophysiological correlates of cognition. In J.E. Desmedt (Ed.), *Cognitive components in cerebral event-related potentials and selective attention.* Progress in Clinical Neurophysiology series, Vol. 6. Basel: Karger.

Cupp, C.J., & Uemura, E. 1980. Age-related changes in prefrontal cortex of Macaca mulatta: Quantitative analysis of dendritic branching patterns. *Experimental Neurology* 69:143-163.

Darlington, R.B., Royce, J.M., Snipper, A.S., Murray, H.W., & Lazar, I. 1981. Preschool programs and later school competence of children from low-income families. *Science* 208:202-204.

Donchin, E. 1981. Surprise!...Surprise? *Psychophysiology* 18:493-513.

Donovick, P.J., & Burright, R.G. 1984. Roots to the future: Gene-environment coaction and individual vulnerability to neural insult. In S. Finger & C.R. Almli (Eds.), *Early brain damage* (Vol. 2). New York: Academic Press.

Douglas, J.W.B. 1975. Early hospital admissions and later disturbances of behavior and learning. *Developmental Medicine and Child Neurology* 17:456-480.

Dreyfus-Brisac, C. 1968. Sleep ontogenesis in early human prematurity from 24 to 27 weeks of conceptional age. *Developmental Psychobiology* 1(3):162-169.

Dreyfus-Brisac, C. 1970. Ontogenesis of brain bioelectrical activity and sleep organization in neonates and infants. In F. Falkner & J.M. Tanner (Eds.), *Human growth.* New York: Plenum Press.

Drillien, C.M. 1974. *The growth and development of the prematurely born infant*. Edinburgh: Livingstone.

Elardo, R., Bradley, R.H., & Caldwell, B. 1977. A longitudinal study of the relation of infants' home environments to language development at age three. *Child Development* 48:595-603.

Emde, R.N., & Koenig, K.L. 1969. Neonatal smiling, frowning, and rapid eye movement states, II Sleep-cycle study. *Journal of Child Psychiatry* 8(4):637-656.

Emde, R.N., & Robinson, J. 1976. The first two months: Recent research in developmental psychobiology and the changing view of the newborn. In J. Noshpitz & J. Call (Eds.), *Basic handbook of child psychiatry*. New York: Basic Books.

Escalona, S. 1963. Patterns of infantile experience and the developmental process. In R. Eissler et al. (Eds.), *The psychoanalytic study of the child* (Vol. 18). New York: International Universities Press.

Escalona, S., Leitch, M., et al. 1952. Early phases of personality development: A non-normative study of infant behavior. *Monographs of the Society for Research in Child Development* 17(1), serial no. 54.

Fahey, J.M. 1986. The hematological effects of the Ca2+ antagonists, nimodipine and verapamil, on sodium nitrite-induced methemoglobinemia. Unpublished master's thesis, University Center at Binghamton, NY.

Feuerstein, R. 1977. Mediated learning experience: A theoretical basis for cognitive human modifiability during adolescence. In P. Mittler (Ed.), *Research to practice in mental retardation* (Vol. 2). Baltimore: University Park Press.

Field, T.M. 1979. Interaction patterns of preterm and term infants. In T.M. Field, A. Sostek, S. Goldberg, & H.H. Shuman (Eds.), *Infants born at risk: Behavior and development*. New York: Spectrum.

Field, T.M., Dempsey, J.R., Hatch, J., Ting, G., & Clifton, R.K. 1979. Cardiac and behavioral responses to repeated tactile and auditory stimulation by preterm and term neonates. *Developmental Psychology* 15:406.

Field, T.M., & Goldson, E. 1984. Pacifying effects of nonnutritive sucking on term and preterm neonates during heelsticks. *Pediatrics* 74:1012-1015.

Field, T.M., Ignatoff, E., Stringer, S., Brennan, J., Greenberg, R., Widmayer, S., & Anderson, G. 1982. Nonnutritive sucking during tube feedings: Effects on preterm neonates in an ICU. *Pediatrics* 70:381-384.

Field, T.M., Schanberg, S.M., Scafidi, F., Bauer, C.R., Vega- Lahr, N., Garcia, R., Nystrom, J., & Kuhn, C.M. 1986. Tactile/kinesthetic stimulation effects on preterm neonates. *Pediatrics* 77:654-658.

Field, T.M., & Sostek, A. 1983. *Infants born at risk: Physiological, perceptual, and cognitive processes.* New York: Grune & Stratton.

Field, T.M., Sostek, A., Goldberg, S., & Shuman, H. (Eds.). 1979. *Infants born at risk: Behavior and development.* New York: Spectrum.

Finkelstein, N.W., & Ramey, C.T. 1980. Information from birth certificate data as a risk index for school failure. *American Journal of Mental Deficiency* 84:546-552.

Fleckenstein, A. 1981. Fundamental actions of calcium antagonists on myocardial and cardiac pacemaker cell membranes. In G.B. Weiss (Ed.), *New perspectives on calcium antagonists.* Bethesda, Md.: American Physiological Society.

Ford, J.M., Mohs, R.C., Pfefferbaum, A., & Kopell, B.S. 1980. On the utility of P3 latency and RT for studying cognitive processes. *Progress in Brain Research* 54:661-667.

Freud, S. 1920. *Beyond the pleasure principle.* Standard ed. 18:7-61. London: Hogarth Press, 1955.

Fuhrmann, P.J. 1984. The effect of preterm infants' state regulation on parent-child interaction. Unpublished master's thesis, University of Washington.

Fukumoto, M., Mochizuki, N., Takeishi, M., Nomura, Y., & Segawa, M. 1981. Studies of body movements during night sleep in infancy. *Brain and Development* 3(1):37-43.

Glass, P., Avery, G.B., Subramanian, K.N.S., Keys, M.P., Sostek, A.M., & Friendly, D.S. 1985. Effect of bright light in the hospital nursery on the incidence of retinopathy of prematurity. *The New England Journal of Medicine* 313:401-404.

Goldberg, S. 1978. Prematurity: Effects on parent-infant interaction. *Journal of Pediatric Psychology* 3:137.

Goldman, P.S., & Nauta, W.J.H. 1977. Columnar distribution of cortico-cortical fibers in the frontal association, limbic, and motor cortex of the developing rhesus monkey. *Brain Research* 122:393-413.

Goldman-Rakic, P.S. 1981. Development and plasticity of primate frontal association cortex. In F.O. Schmitt, F.G. Worden, S.G. Dennis, & G. Adelman (Eds.), *The organization of the cerebral cortex.* Cambridge, Mass.: MIT Press.

Goldman-Rakic, P.S., Isseroff, A., Schwartz, M.L., & Bugbee, N.M. 1983. The neurobiology of cognitive development. In P. Mussen (Ed.), *Handbook of child psychology: Biology and infancy development.* New York: Wiley.

Goldman-Rakic, P.S., & Schwartz, M.L. 1982. Interdigitation of contralateral and ipsilateral columnar projections to frontal association cortex in primates. *Science* 216:755-757.

Goodin, D.S., Squires, K.C., & Starr, A. 1978. Long latency event-related components of the auditory evoked potentials in dementia. *Brain* 101:635-648.

Gorski, P., and colleagues. 1984. Caring for immature infants—A touchy subject. In C. Brown (Ed.), *The many facets of touch.* Skillman, N.J.: Johnson & Johnson Baby Products Company.

Gorski, P.A., Hole, W.T., Leonard, C.H., & Martin, J.A. 1983. Direct computer recording of premature infants and nursery care: Distress following two interventions. *Pediatrics* 72:198-202.

Gottfried, A.W. (Ed.). 1984. *Home environment and early cognitive development: Longitudinal research.* Orlando, Fla.: Academic Press.

Gottfried, A.W., & Gaiter, J.L. 1985. *Infant stress under intensive care.* Baltimore: University Park Press.

Gottfried, A.W., Wallace-Lande, P., Sherman-Brown, S., King, J., Coen, C., & Hodgman, J.E. 1981. Physical and social environment of newborn infants in special care units. *Science* 214:673-675.

Gottlieb, G. 1971a. *Development of species identification in birds.* Chicago: University of Chicago Press.

Gottlieb, G. 1971b. Ontogenesis of sensory function in birds and mammals. In E. Tobach, L.R. Aronson, & E. Shaw (Eds.), *The biopsychology of development.* New York: Academic Press.

Gottlieb, G. 1976. Conceptions of prenatal development: Behavioral embryology. *Psychological Review* 83(3):215-234.

Graham, F.K., & Clifton, R.K. 1966. Heart rate change as a component of the orienting response. *Psychological Bulletin* 65:305-320.

Grant, V.J. 1983. Pedestrian traffic in a pediatric ward. *New Zealand Medical Journal* 96:91-93.

Gunnar, M.R., Isensee, J., & Fust, S. In press. Adrenocorticol activity and the Brazelton Neonatal Assessment Scale: Moderating effects of the newborn's biobehavioral status. *Child Development*.

Hagemann, V. 1981a. Night sleep of children in a hospital, part 1: Sleep duration. *Maternal-Child Nursing Journal* 10:1-13.

Hagemann, V. 1981b. Night sleep of children in a hospital, part 2: Sleep disruption. *Maternal-Child Nursing Journal* 10:127-142.

Hardy, C. 1985. The behavioral and physiological consequences of right middle cerebral artery ligation in rats following treatment with nimodipine, a calcium voltage-operated channel blocker. Unpublished doctoral dissertation, University Center at Binghamton, N.Y.

Harlow, H.F. 1958. The nature of love. *American Psychologist* 13:673-685.

Hebb, D.O. 1949. *The organization of behavior.* New York: Wiley.

Hecox, K. 1975. Electrophysiological correlates of human auditory development. In L. Cohen & P. Salapatek (Eds.), *Infant perception* (Vol. 2). New York: Academic Press.

Heistad, D.D., & Haws, C.W. 1985. Effects of nimodipine in cerebral blood flow and cerebral vasoconstrictor responses: Implications for membrane mechanisms. In E. Betz, K. Deck, & F. Hoffmeister (Eds.), *Nimodipine: Pharmacological and clinical properties. Proceedings of the First International Nimotop Symposium* (pp. 47-53). New York: F.K. Schattauer-Verlag.

High, P.C., & Gorski, P.A. 1985. Womb for improvement—Recording environmental influences on infant development in the intensive care nursery. In A.W. Gottfried & J.L. Gaiter (Eds.), *Infant stress under intensive care: Environmental neonatology.* Baltimore: University Park Press.

Hoffmeister, F., Benz, V., Heise, A., Krause, H.P., & Neuser, V. 1982. Behavioral effects of nimodipine in animals. *Arzneimittel-Forschung/Drug Research* 32:347-360.

Horowitz, F.D. In press. *Exploring developmental theories: Toward a structural/behavioral model* (tentative title). Hillsdale, N.J.: Erlbaum.

Howard, J., Parmelee, A.H., Jr., Kopp, C.B., & Littman, B. 1976. A neurologic comparison of pre-term and full-term infants at term conceptual age. *Journal of Pediatrics* 88:995-1002.

Hubel, D.H., & Wiesel, T.N. 1977. Functional architecture of macaque monkey visual cortex. *Proceedings of the Royal Society of London.* B. 193:1-59.

Hunt, J.McV. 1961. *Intelligence and experience.* New York: Ronald Press.

Innocenti, G.M. 1981. Growth and reshaping of axons in the establishment of visual callosal connections. *Science* 212:824-827.

Innocenti, G.M., & Clarke, S. 1984. Bilateral transitory projection to visual areas from auditory cortex in kittens. *Developmental Brain Research* 14:143-148.

Innocenti, G.M., Frost, D.F., & Illes, J. 1985. Maturation of visual callosal connections in visually deprived kittens: A challenging critical period. *Journal of Neuroscience* 5:255-267.

Isaacson, R.L. 1982. *The limbic system.* 2d ed. New York: Plenum Press.

Isaacson, R.L., Springer, J.E., & Ryan, J.P. 1986. Cholinergic and catecholaminergic modification of the hippocampal lesion syndrome. In R.L. Isaacson & K.H. Pribram (Eds.), *The hippocampus* (Vol. 4). New York: Plenum Press.

Iuvone, P.M., & Van Hartesveldt, C. 1976. Locomotor activity and plasma corticosterone in rats with hippocampal lesions. *Behavioral Biology* 16:515-520.

Ivy, G.O., & Killackey, H.P. 1982. Ontogenetic changes in the projections of neocortical neurons. *Journal of Neuroscience* 2:735-743.

Jacobson, S., & Trojanowski, J.Q. 1977a. Prefrontal granular cortex of the rhesus monkey. I. Intrahemispheric cortical afferents. *Brain Research* 132:209-233.

Jacobson, S., & Trojanowski, J.Q. 1977b. Prefrontal granular cortex of the rhesus monkey. II. Interhemispheric cortical afferents. *Brain Research* 132:235-246.

Jay, S. 1982. The effects of gentle human touch on mechanically ventilated very short gestation infants. *Maternal-Child Nursing Journal* 11:199-256.

Jensen, A.R. 1969. How much can we boost IQ and scholastic achievement? *Harvard Educational Review* 39:1-123.

Kang, R., & Barnard, K.E. 1979. Using the Neonatal Behavioral Assessment Scale to evaluate premature infants. In *Birth defects: Original article series* (Vol. 15) 7:119-144. New York: Alan R. Liss.

Karnes, M.B. 1975. *GOAL program: Mathematical concepts.* Springfield, Mass.: Milton-Bradley.

Kazda, S., & Hoffmeister, F. 1979. Effect of some cerebral dilators on the post-ischemic impaired cerebral reperfusion in cats. *Archives of Pharmacology* 307, R43.

Korner, A.F. 1964. Some hypotheses regarding the significance of individual differences at birth for later development. In R. Eissler et al. (Eds.), *The psychoanalytic study of the child* (Vol. 19). New York: International Universities Press.

Korner, A.F. 1969. Neonatal startles, smiles, erections, and reflex sucks as related to state, sex, and individuality. *Child Development* 40(4):1039-1053.

Korner, A.F. 1971. Individual differences at birth: Implications for early experience and later development. *American Journal of Orthopsychiatry* 41(4):609-618.

Korner, A.F. 1972. State as variable, as obstacle and as mediator of stimulation in infant research. *Merrill-Palmer Quarterly* 18(2):77-94.

Korner, A.F. 1981. What we don't know about water beds and apneic preterm infants (letter). *Pediatrics* 68(2):306-307.

Korner, A.F. 1986. *Neurobehavioral maturity assessment for preterm infants.* Unpublished manuscript.

Korner, A.F., Guilleminault, C., Vanden Hoed, J., & Baldwin, R.B. 1978. Reduction of sleep apnea and bradycardia in preterm infants on oscillation waterbeds: A controlled polygraphic study. *Pediatrics* 61(4):528-533.

Korner, A.F., Hutchinson, C.A., Koperski, J., Kraemer, H.C., & Schneider, P.A. 1981. Stability of individual differences of neonatal motor and crying patterns. *Child Development* 52:83-90.

Korner, A.F., Kraemer, H.C., Haffner, M.E., & Cosper, L. 1975. Effects of waterbed flotation on premature infants: A pilot study. *Pediatrics* 56(3):361-367.

Korner, A.F., Schneider, P., & Forrest, T. 1983. Effects of vestibular-proprioceptive stimulation on the neurobehavioral development of preterm infants: A pilot study. *Neuropediatrics* 14(3):170-175.

Korner, A.F., Zeanah, C.H., Linden, J., Kraemer, H.C., Berkowitz, R.I., & Agras, W.S. 1985. Relation between neonatal and later activity and temperament. *Child Development* 56(1):38-42.

Krafchuk, E.E., Tronick, E.Z., & Clifton, R.K. 1983. Behavioral and cardiac responses to sound in preterm neonates varying in risk status: A hypothesis of their paradoxical reactivity. In T.M. Field & A. Sostek (Eds.), *Infants born at risk: Physiological, perceptual, and cognitive processes.* New York: Grune & Stratton.

Krech, D., Rosenzweig, M.R., & Bennett, E.L. 1960. Effects of early environmental complexity and training on brain chemistry. *Journal of Comparative and Physiological Psychology* 53:509-519.

Krumholz, A., Felinx, J.K., Goldstein, P.J., & McKenzie, E. 1985. Maturation of the brain-stem auditory evoked potential in premature infants. *Electroencephalography and Clinical Neurophysiology* 62:124-134.

Lawson, K., Daum, C., & Turkewitz, G. 1977. Environmental characteristics of a neonatal intensive care unit. *Child Development* 48:1633-1639.

Lester, B. 1983. Change and stability in neonatal behavior. In T.B. Brazelton & B.M. Lester (Eds.), *New approaches to developmental screening of infants.* New York: Elsevier.

Lester, B.M., Als, H., & Brazelton, T.B. 1982. Regional obstetric anesthesia and newborn behavior: A reanalysis toward synergistic effects. *Child Development* 53:687-692.

Lester, B.M., Emory, E.K., & Hoffman, S.L. 1976. A multivariate study of the effects of high-risk factors on performance on the Brazelton Neonatal Assessment Scale. *Child Development* 47:515-517.

Lester, B.M., Hoffman, J., & Brazelton, T.B. 1984. The rhythmic structure of mother-infant interaction in term and preterm infants. *Child Development* 56:15-28.

Lindeman, E. 1944. Grief. *American Journal of Psychology* 101:141.

Linn, P.L., & Horowitz, F.D. 1983. The relationship between infant individual differences & mother-infant interaction during the neonatal period. *Infant Behavior and Development* 6:415-427.

Long, J.G., Alistair, G.S., Philip, A.G.S., & Lucey, J.F. 1980. Excessive handling as a cause of hypoxemia. *Pediatrics* 65:203-206.

Lorenz, K. 1937. Companion in the bird's world. *Auk* 54:245-273.

McQuiston, S. 1982. Mother-infant interaction in infants with Down syndrome. *Dissertation Abstracts International* 42:4534A-4535A (University Microfilms no. 82-38).

Meijer, A. 1985. Hospitalization in infancy as a long-term at-risk indicator. In S. Harel & N.J. Anastasiow (Eds.), *The at-risk infant: Psycho/social/medical aspects*. Baltimore: Brooks.

Miller, N.E. 1959. Liberalization of basic S-R concepts: Extensions to conflict behavior, motivation and social learning. In S. Koch (Ed.), *Psychology: A study of a science* (Vol. 2). New York: McGraw-Hill.

Milliones, J. 1978. Relationships between perceived child temperament and maternal behaviors. *Child Development* 49:1255.

Monod, N., & Garma, L. 1971. Auditory responsivity in the human premature. *Biology of the Neonate* 17:292-316.

Morrison-Graham, K. 1983. An anatomical and electrophysiological study of synapse elimination at the developing frog neuromuscular junction. *Developmental Biology* 99:298-311.

Neal, M.V. 1967. The relationship between a regimen of vestibular stimulation and the developmental behavior of the premature infant. *Dissertation Abstracts International* (University Microfilms no. 70-7342).

Nurcombe, B., Howell, D.C., Rauh, V.A., Teti, D.M., Ruoff, P., & Brennan, J. 1984. An intervention program for mothers of low-birthweight infants: Preliminary results. *Journal of the American Academy of Child Psychiatry* 23:319-325.

Nurcombe, B., Rauh, V., Howell, D.C., Teti, D.M., Ruoff, P., Murphy, B., & Brennan, J. 1984. An intervention program for mothers of low-birthweight babies: Outcome at six and twelve months. In J.D. Call, E. Galenson, & R.L. Tyson (Eds.), *Frontiers of Infant Psychiatry*. New York: Basic Books.

Nyakas, C.S., De Kloet, E.R., Veldhuis, H.D., & Bohus, B. 1983. Hippocampal corticosterone receptors and novelty-induced behavioral activity: Effect of kainic acid lesions in the hippocampus. *Brain Research* 288:219-228.

O'Leary, D.D.M., Stanfield, B.B., & Cowan, W.M. 1981. Evidence that the early postnatal restriction of the cells of origin of the callosal projection is due to the elimination of axonal collaterals rather than to the death of neurons. *Developmental Brain Research* 1:607-617.

Papile, L.A., Burstein, J., Burstein, R., & Koffler, H. 1978. Incidence and evolution of subependymal and intraventricular hemorrhage: A study of infants with birth weights less than 1,500 grams. *Journal of Pediatrics* 92(4):529-534.

Papile, L.A., Munsick-Bruno, G., & Schaefer, A. 1983. Relationship of cerebral intraventricular hemorrhage and early childhood neurologic handicaps. *Journal of Pediatrics* 103(2):273-277.

Parmelee, A.H., Jr., Sigman, M., Kopp, C.B., & Haber, A. 1975. The concept of a cumulative risk score for infants. In N.R. Ellis (Ed.), *Aberrant development in infancy: Human and animal studies.* Hillsdale, N.J.: Erlbaum.

Parmelee, A.H., Jr., & Stern, E. 1972. Development of states in infants. In C.D. Clemente, D.P. Purpura, & F.E. Mayer (Eds.), *Sleep and the maturing nervous system.* New York: Academic Press.

Paton, J.A., & Nottebohm, F.N. 1984. Neurons generated in the adult brain are recruited into functional circuits. *Science* 225:1046-1048.

Peirano, P., Curze-Dascalova, L., Korn, G., & Vincente, G. 1986. Influence of sleep state and age on body motility in normal premature and full-term neonates. *Neopediatrics* 17:186-190.

Penfield, W.G., & Boldrey, E. 1937. Somatic motor and sensory representation in the cerebral cortex of man as studied by electrical stimulation. *Brain* 60:389.

Pfefferbaum, A.J., Ford, J.M., Roth, W.T., & Kopell, B.S. 1980. Age-related changes in auditory event-related potentials. *Electroencephalography and Clinical Neurophysiology* 49:266-276.

Piaget, J. 1952. *The Origins of Intelligence in Children.* 2d ed. New York: International Universities Press.

Picton, T.W., Stuss, D.T., Champagne, S.C., & Nelson, R.F. 1984. The effects of age on human event-related potentials. *Psychophysiology* 21:312-325.

Porges, S.W., McCabe, P.M., & Yongue, B.G. 1982. Respiratory—heart rate interactions: Psychophysiological implications for pathophysiology and behavior. In J. Caccioppo & R. Petty (Eds.), *Perspectives in cardiovascular psychophysiology.* New York: Gilford.

Prechtl, H.F.R., & Beintema, D.J. 1964. *The neurological examination of the full-term infant.* Clinics in developmental medicine, no. 12. Philadelphia: Spastics Society with Heinemann.

Prechtl, H.F.R. 1968. Neurological findings in newborn infants after pre- and perinatal complications. In *Aspects of prematurity and dysmaturity*, Nutrica Symposium, Gronigen, 1967. Leiden: H.E. Stenfert Kroese N.V.

Prechtl, H.F.R. 1974. The behavioural states of the newborn infant (a review). *Brain Research* 76:185-212.

Prechtl, H.F.R., Fargel, J.W., Weinmann, H.M., & Bakker, H.H. 1979. Postures, motility and respiration of low-risk pre-term infants. *Developmental Medicine and Child Neurology* 21:3-27.

Pujol, R., & Hilding, D. 1973. Anatomy and physiology of the onset of auditory function. *Acta Oto-laryngologica* (Basel) 76:1-10.

Quinton, D., & Rutter, M. 1976. Early hospital admissions and later disturbances of behaviour: An attempted replication of Douglas' findings. *Developmental Medicine and Child Neurology* 18:447-459.

Ramey, C.T., & Bryant, D.M. 1982. Evidence for prevention of developmental retardation during infancy. *Journal of the Division for Early Childhood* 5:73-78.

Ramey, C.T., Bryant, D.M., & Suarez, T.M. In press. Preschool compensatory education and the modifiability of intelligence: A critical review. In Detterman (Ed.), *Current topics in human intelligence.* Norwood, N.J.: Ablex.

Ramey, C.T., & MacPhee, D. In press. Developmental retardation among the poor: A systems theory perspective on risk and prevention. In D.C. Farran & J.D. McKinney (Eds.), *Risk in intellectual and psychosocial development.* Orlando, Fla.: Academic Press.

Ramey, C.T., MacPhee, D., & Yeates, K.O. 1982. Preventing developmental retardation: A general systems model. In L. Bond & J. Joffe (Eds.), *Facilitating infant and early childhood development.* Hanover, N.H.: University Press of New England.

Ramey, C.T., Sparling, J.J., Bryant, D.M., & Wasik, B.H. 1982. Primary prevention of developmental retardation during infancy. *Prevention in Human Services* 1:61-83. Reprinted in H.A. Moss, R. Moss, & C. Swift (Eds.), *Early intervention programs for infants.* New York: Haworth Press.

Ramey, C.T., Trohanis, P.L., & Hostler, S.L. 1982. An Introduction. In C.T. Ramey & P.L. Trohanis (Eds.), *Finding and educating high-risk and handicapped infants.* Baltimore: University Park Press.

Ramey, C.T., Yeates, K.O., & Short, E.J. 1984. The plasticity of intellectual development: Insights from preventive intervention. *Child Development* 55:1913-1925.

Rauh, V., Achenbach, T., Nurcombe, B., Howell, D.C., & Teti, D. Overcoming neonatal adversity: Four-year results of an intervention for low-birthweight infants. Manuscript submitted for publication.

Reinstein, D.K., Hannigan, J.H., Jr., & Isaacson, R.L. 1982. Time course of certain behavioral changes after hippocampal damage and their alteration by dopaminergic intervention into nucleus accombens. *Pharmacology, Biochemistry, and Behavior* 17:193-202.

Richards, J.E. 1987. Infant visual sustained attention and respiratory sinus arrhythmia. *Child Development* 58:488-496.

Rothblat, L.A., & Schwartz, M.L. 1978. Altered early environment: Affects on the brain and visual behavior. In R.D. Walk & H.L. Pick (Eds.), *Perception and experience*. New York: Plenum Press.

Rothchild, B.T. 1966. Incubator isolation as a possible continuating factor to the high incidence of emotional disturbance among premature born persons. *Journal of Genetic Psychology* 110:287-304.

Ryan, J.R., Springer, J.E., Hannigan, J.H., Jr., & Isaacson, R.L. 1985. Suppression of corticosterone synthesis alters the behavior of hippocampally lesioned rats. *Behavioral and Neural Biology* 44:47-59.

Salamy, A., & McKean, C.M. 1976. Postnatal development of human brainstem potentials during the first year of life. *Electroencephalography and Clinical Neurophysiology* 40:418-426.

Salamy, A., McKean, C.M., Pettett, G., & Mendelson, T. 1978. Auditory brainstem recovery processes from birth to adulthood. *Psychophysiology* 15:214-220.

Sameroff, A.J., & Chandler, M.J. 1975. Reproductive risk and the continuum of care-taking casualty. In F.D. Horowitz (Ed.), *Review of child development research* (Vol. 4). Chicago: University of Chicago Press.

Scanlon, K., Scanlon, J., & Tronick, E. 1984. The impact of perinatal and neonatal events on the early behavior of the extremely premature human. *Journal of Developmental and Behavioral Pediatrics* 5:65-73.

Schanberg, S.M., Evoniuk, G., & Kuhn, C. 1984. Tactile and nutritional aspects of maternal care: Specific regulators of neuroendocrine function and cellular development. *Proceedings of the Society for Experimental Biology and Medicine* 175:135-146.

Schanberg, S.M., & Field, T.M. In press. Sensory deprivation stress and supplemental stimulation in the rat pup and the preterm human neonate. *Child Development.*

Scheibel, A.B., & Tomiyasu, U. 1978. Dendritic sprouting in Alzheimer's presenile dementia. *Experimental Neurology* 60:1-8.

Scheibel, M.E., & Scheibel, A.B. 1958. Structural substrates for integrative patterns in the brain stem reticular core. In H.H. Jaspar, L.D. Proctor, R.S. Knighton, W.C. Noshay, & R.T. Costello (Eds.), *Reticular formation of the brain.* Boston: Little Brown.

Schwartz, M.L., & Goldman-Rakic, P.S. 1984. Callosal and intrahemispheric connectivity of the prefrontal association cortex in rhesus monkey: Relation between intraparietal and principal sulcal cortex. *Journal of Comparative Neurology* 226:403-420.

Scriabine, A., Battye, R., Hoffmeister, F., Kazda, S., Towart, R., Garthoff, B., Schluter, G., Ramsch, K., & Scherling, D. 1985. Nimodipine. In A. Scriabine (Ed.), *New drugs annal: Cardiovascular drugs.* New York: Raven Press.

Sell, E., Luick, A., & Poisson, S. 1980. Outcome of very low birthweight infants. 1. Neonatal behavior of 188 infants. *Journal of Developmental and Behavioral Pediatrics* 1:78-82.

Shea, E., & Tronick, E.Z. In press. The maternal self-report inventory: A research and clinical instrument for assessing maternal self-esteem. In H.E. Fitzgerald, B. Lester, & M.W. Yogman (Eds.), *Theory and Research in Behavioral Pediatrics* (Vol. 4). New York: Plenum Press.

Siegel, L.S. 1982a. Reproductive, perinatal and environmental variables as predictors of development of preterm (1501 grams) and full-term children at 5 years. *Seminars in Perinatology* 6:274-279.

Siegel, L.S. 1982b. Reproductive, perinatal and environmental factors as predictors of the cognitive and language development of preterm and full-term infants. *Child Development* 53:963-973.

Siegel, L.S. 1985. Biological and environmental variables as predictors of intellectual functioning at 6 years of age. In S. Harel & N.J. Anastasiow (Eds.), *The at-risk infant: Psycho/social/medical aspects.* Baltimore: Brooks.

Siegel, L.S., Saigal, S., Rosenbaum, P., Morton, R.A., Young, A., Berenbaum, S., & Stoskopf, B. 1982. Predictors of development in preterm and fullterm infants: A model for detecting the at-risk child. *Journal of Pediatric Psychology* 1:135-148.

Skeels, H.M. 1966. Adult status of children with contrasting early life experiences. *Monographs of the Society for Research in Child Development* 31(3), serial no. 105.

Skeels, H.M., Updegraff, R., Wellman, B.L., & Williams, H.L. 1938. A study of environmental stimulation: An orphanage preschool project. *University of Iowa Studies in Child Welfare* (Vol. 15, no. 4).

Smith, J.C. 1976. Spending time with the hospitalized child. *MCN: American Journal of Maternal Child Nursing* 1:164.

Sostek, A.M., Quinn, P.O., & Davitt, M.X. 1979. Behavior, development and neurologic status of premature and full-term infants with varying medical complications. In T.M. Field (Ed.), *Infants born at risk: Behavior and development*. New York: Spectrum.

Spinelli, D.N. 1967. Receptive field organization of ganglion cells in the cat's retina. *Experimental Neurology* 19:291-315.

Spinelli, D.N., Hirsch, H.V., Phelps, R.W., & Metzler, J. 1972. Visual experience as a determinant of the response characteristics of cortical receptive fields in cats. *Experimental Brain Research* 15:289-304.

Spinelli, D.N., & Jensen, F.E. 1979. Plasticity: The mirror of experience. *Science* 203:75-79.

Spinelli, D.N., & Jensen, F.E. 1982. Plasticity, experience, and resource allocation in motor cortex and hypothalamus. In C.D. Woody (Ed.), *Conditioning*. New York: Plenum Press.

Spitz, R. 1965. *The first year of life: Normal and deviant object relations*. New York: International Universities Press.

Springer, J.E., & Isaacson, R.L. 1982. Catecholamine alterations in basal ganglia after hippocampal lesions. *Brain Research* 252:185-188.

Springer, J.E., Ryan, J.R., & Isaacson, R.L. Acute choline administration produces transient reductions in the effects of hippocampal destruction. Unpublished paper.

Squires, K.C., Donchin, E., Herning, R., & McCarthy, G. 1977. On the influence of task relevance and stimulus probability on ERP components. *Electroencephalography and Clinical Neurophysiology* 42:1-14.

Squires, K.C., Wickens, C., Squires, N.K., & Donchin, E. 1976. The effect of stimulus sequence in the waveform of the cortical event-related potential. *Science* 193:1142-1146.

Starr, A., Amlie, R.N., Martin, W.H.J., & Sanders, S. 1977. Development of auditory function in newborn infants revealed by auditory brainstem potentials. *Pediatrics* 60:831-839.

Stern, D.N. 1974. Mother and infant at play: The dyadic interaction involving facial, vocal and gaze behaviors. In M. Lewis & L.A. Rosenblum (Eds.), *The origins of behavior.* Vol. 1, *The effect of the infant on its caregiver.* New York: Wiley.

Stubbe, P., & Wolf, H. 1971. The effect of stress on growth hormone, glucose and glycerol levels in newborn infants. *Hormones and Metabolic Research* 3:175-179.

Syndulko, K., Hansch, E.C., Cohen, S.N., Pearce, J.W., Goldberg, Z., Montan, B., Tourtelotte, W.W., & Potvin, A.R. 1982. Long-latency event related potentials in normal aging and dementia. In J. Courjon, R. Mauguiere, & M. Revol (Eds.), *Clinical applications of evoked potentials in neurology.* New York: Raven Press.

Telzrow, R.W., Kang, R., Mitchell, S.K., Ashworth, C.D., & Barnard, K.E. 1982. An assessment of the behavior of the premature infant of forty weeks conceptional age. In L.P. Lipsitt & T.M. Field (Eds.), *Perinatal risk and newborn behavior.* Norwood, N.J.: Ablex.

Thoman, E.B., Acebo, C., Dreyer, C.A., Becker, P.T., & Freese, M.P. 1979. Individuality and the interactive process. In E.B. Thoman (Ed.), *Origins of the infant's social responsiveness.* Hillsdale, N.J.: Erlbaum.

Thoman, E.B., & Becker, P.T. 1979. Issues in assessment and prediction for the infant born at risk. In T.M. Field et al. (Eds.), *Infants born at risk: Behavior and development.* New York: Spectrum.

Thoman, E.B., Miano, V.N., & Freese, M.P. 1977. The role of respiratory instability in the Sudden Infant Death Syndrome. *Developmental Medicine and Child Neurology* 19:729-738.

Thompson, W.R., & Heron, W. 1954. The effects of early restriction on activity in dogs. *Journal of Comparative and Physiological Psychology* 47:77-82.

Towbin, A. 1970. Central nervous system damage in the human fetus and newborn infant. *American Journal of Diseases of Children* 119:529-542.

Tronick, E., & Brazelton, T.B. 1975. Clinical uses of the Brazelton Neonatal Behavior Assessment. In B.Z. Friedlander, G.B. Sterritt, & G.E. Kirk (Eds.), *Exceptional infant* (Vol. 3). New York: Brunner/Mazel.

Tronick, E.Z., Scanlon, K., & Scanlon, J. In press. Behavioral organization and its relation to clinical and physiological status of the preterm infant during the newborn period: Apathetic organization may not be abnormal. In B. Lester, & E.Z. Tronick (Eds.), *In defense of the premature infant: The limits of plasticity.* Lexington, Mass.: Lexington Books.

Tynan, W.D. 1986. Behavioral stability predicts morbidity and mortality in infants from a neonatal intensive care unit. *Infant Behavior and Development* 9:71-79.

Wagner, M., & McCue, K. 1987. Collaborative approaches to research with hospitalized infants. Paper presented at 22d Annual Conference of Association for the Care of Children's Health, Halifax, Nova Scotia.

Watanabe, K., Iwase, K., & Hara, K. 1973. Heart rate variability during sleep and wakefulness in low-birthweight infants. *Biology of the Neonate* 22:87-98.

Wecker, L., & Dettbarn, W.D. 1979. Relationship between choline availability and acetylcholine synthesis in discrete regions of rat brain. *Journal of Neurochemistry* 32:961-967.

Wecker, L., Dettbarn, W.D., & Schmidt, D.E. 1978. Choline administration: Modification of the central actions of atropine. *Science* 199:86-87.

Wieloch, T. 1985. Neurochemical correlates to selective neuronal vulnerability. *Progress in Brain Research* 63:69-85.

Wolff, P.H. 1966. The causes, controls, and organization of behavior in the neonate. *Psychological Issues*, Vol. 5, no. 1, monograph 17. New York: International Universities Press.

Yeates, I.O., MacPhee, D., Campbell, F.A., & Ramey, C.T. 1983. Maternal IQ and home environment as determinants of early childhood intellectual competence: A developmental analysis. *Developmental Psychology* 19(5):731-739.

Zeskind, P.S., & Ramey, C.T. 1978. Fetal malnutrition: An experimental study of its consequences on infants in two caregiving environments. *Child Development* 49:1155-1162.

Zeskind, P.S., & Ramey, C.T. 1981. Preventing intellectual and interactional sequelae of fetal malnutrition: A longitudinal, transactional and synergistic approach to development. *Child Development* 52:213-218.